M000188371

The Australian
Healthy
Hormone
DIET

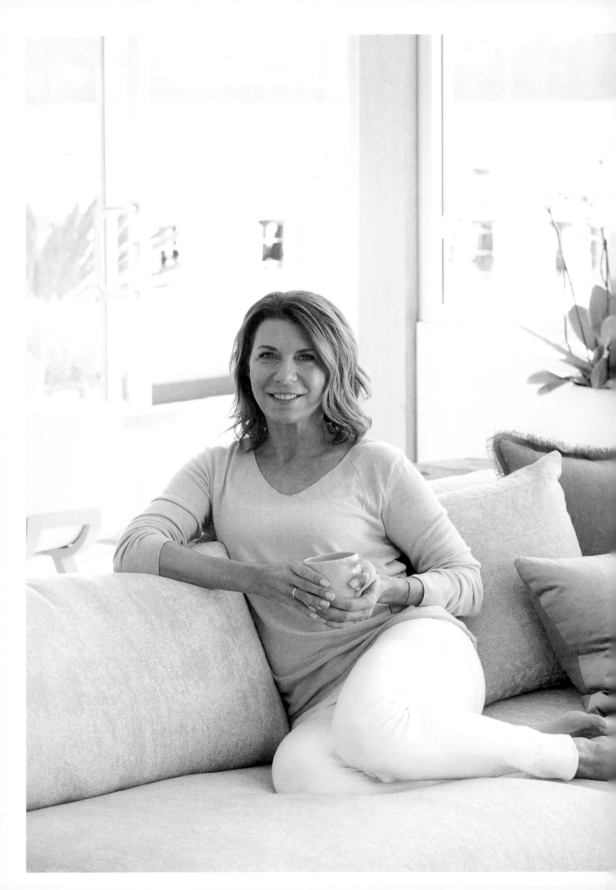

The Australian
Healthy
Hormone
DIET

A 4-week reset with **recipes** and eating plans to help reduce **weight**, increase **energy** and improve **mood**

MICHELE
CHEVALLEY
HEDGE

WITH JENNIFER FLEMING

Pan Macmillan Australia

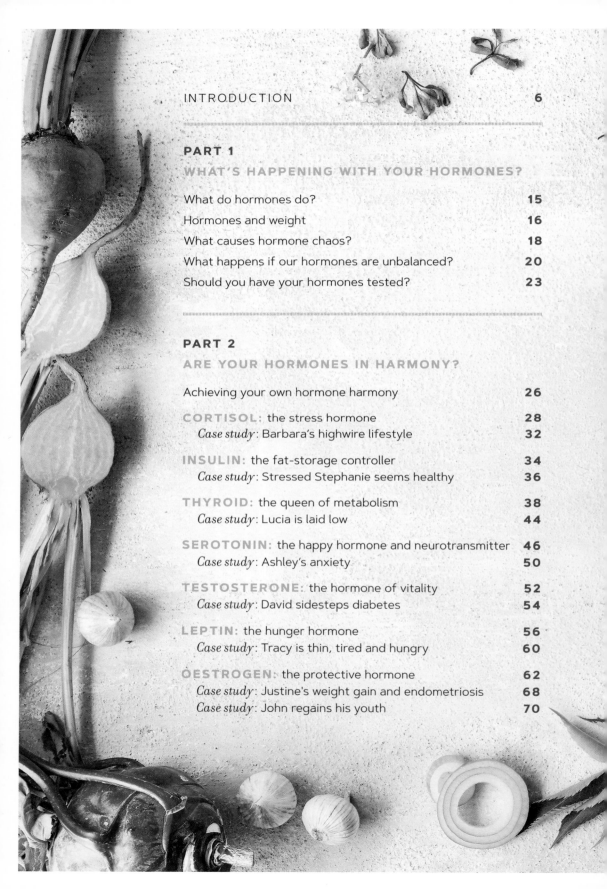

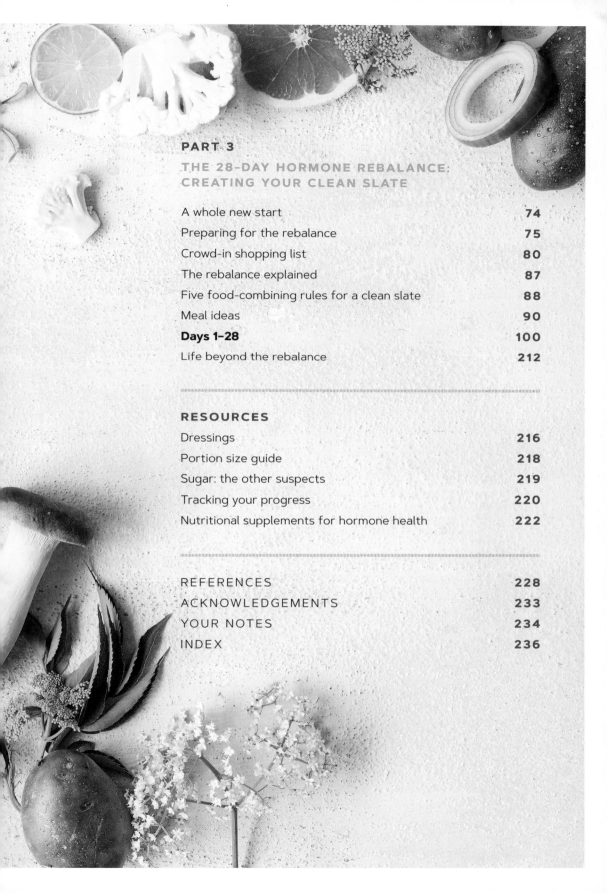

PART 3
THE 28-DAY HORMONE REBALANCE: CREATING YOUR CLEAN SLATE

RESOURCES

INTRODUCTION

Do you feel like you're carrying extra kilos, even though you watch what you eat? How about the exhaustion you feel at the end of the day and sometimes when you wake up?

Do your moods fluctuate over the course of a day, week or month? Do you have a low-level nagging feeling that something just isn't right? Yes, you're able to get on with your busy life, but you feel as though every day is about reaching a finishing line or pushing a rock up a hill.

When did life get this exhausting? You leave the office but work continues, courtesy of your phone. You're tricked into spending too much time with it. You grab it. Time stops. Tap the screen. Punch out an email. Send a text. Check the internet, news, social media. Oh, wait, what's this? What did you want again? Hello, multi-tasking. Frantic families ferry children through congested cities for netball, piano lessons or taekwondo. You spend time with ageing parents. You try to stay connected with busy friends. But what about you? When do you have time for your own health?

Finding time to eat healthy food, exercise, sleep well and release stress is a challenge. When time is one of your most valuable commodities, it's common to take shortcuts or use pick-me-ups to keep you moving. A morning boost with a takeaway coffee. A carb or sugar hit during a mid-afternoon slump.

A seductive glass of wine or three to wind down in the evening. You often eat lunch at your desk – or 'al desko' – a term so frequently used it was added to the Oxford Dictionary in 2014. It's easy to fall into a grab-and-go routine – for you and your family. On the surface, you look like you're coping quite well. But it's more difficult to see what's going on inside your body – and in particular with your hormones.

I'm a qualified nutritionist with my own private practice, A Healthy View. I began running cleanse retreats in 2005, and shortly after that opened my first clinic. Since then, people have seen me for a range of reasons: they want to lose weight; improve their sleep; gain more energy; feel better; or fix their addictions to food. I hear stories of frustration, exhaustion, dissatisfaction and sometimes pain. And more and more, I see clients whose problems are linked to hormone imbalances. When I tell them the reason they feel depleted and exhausted is that their hormone levels are too high or too low, most are surprised. Aside from teenage mood swings, menstruation or menopause, they have no idea how hormones influence how we look and feel. But hormones play an integral part in most vital bodily functions, from growth and metabolism to libido, healthy blood sugar levels and distribution of fat.

WHAT CAUSES HORMONE CHAOS?

It's easy to fall into hormone chaos. Our hormone levels are affected by eating processed sugary foods, poor sleep patterns, bad gut bacteria, the way we deal with stress, and exposure to pollution and chemicals used in plastics, cosmetics and cleaning products. It's common to have more than one hormone out of whack – creating a domino effect. Endocrine disruption, the process by which natural and synthetic chemicals interfere with our hormones, could be one of the main reasons for obesity, diabetes, a sluggish thyroid and reduced fertility.

This book outlines the nutritional and lifestyle changes I use to rebalance my clients' hormones. You should consult your GP or health professional before engaging in these changes. While in some cases you may also need to see an endocrinologist for specialist advice, for many people, simple changes in their diet and lifestyle are enough to restore hormone harmony.

MY OWN STORY OF HORMONE CHAOS

I know what it's like to climb into the hamster wheel every day and run. In a former life I worked as a marketing manager

Stop beating yourself up. Maybe it's not your lack of willpower; maybe it's your hormones. An imbalance of insulin, cortisol, thyroid hormone, serotonin, leptin and oestrogen can make us feel tired, moody and fat.

for Microsoft. I have three children and a husband who frequently travels for work. When I worked in marketing I often felt puffy, with a head full of cotton wool and negative self-talk. Every week my weight fluctuated by 1 to 3 kilograms and was slowly climbing. Clothes in my wardrobe ranged from size 8 to size 16 – and I'm not exaggerating. My digestion was backed up. I was sleeping fewer than seven hours a night and this showed in my skin, mood and weight. I gave a good impression of being on top of things, but inside I was a ball of anxiety and negativity. I remember one morning, after squishing into a tight skirt and blouse, I couldn't bear to look at myself in the mirror to put on my mascara. I moved my body to one side and tilted my head so I could only see one eye at a time. This negative, self-sabotaging behaviour continued for nearly a year.

I've always struggled with my weight. I grew up in a house where food equalled love. For years I used exercise to compensate for all my eating wrongs. If I inhaled half a packet of Tim Tams, I had to run for at least 15 kilometres. While I was usually a healthy eater, rather than eating one serving of yoghurt before bed, I'd eat two – sometimes with a handful of nuts. I often ate three handfuls of nuts. I usually had two avocados in one sitting. You get the picture. The quantities were too large. What can I say? I like food. But however 'healthy' they were, those calories still turned into excess weight. And excess weight was a burden on my mental and emotional state. So I made a conscious choice. I tackled my portion sizes and named them for what they were – portion distortion.

The impact of hormone imbalance didn't really hit me until 2013. That year my brother Greg was diagnosed with a rare form of stage 4 lung cancer. Greg was a fire fighter in New York City, where we grew up, and was one of the first responders following the attack on the World Trade Center on 11 September

2001. Photos of the site after the attack show burnt-out ruins and a thick grey haze. We now know that haze was filled with carcinogenic material, inhaled by my brother and many other first responders.

From the moment Greg was diagnosed in August 2013, every six weeks or so I flew from Sydney to New York City to be his health advocate. I pushed, cajoled and screamed my way through the New York medical system. Greg was a George Clooney lookalike and felt bulletproof to me. Everyone loved him. He was the guy who made you laugh. He built his house himself and started a family with wife Lisa and twin boys, Cooper and Ryder, born in 2012. Greg was a fighter to the end. I can still remember when the oncologists told him his treatment would stop. Greg said, 'I've got two babies. I've just started living. Are you telling me that's it?' He died on 24 April 2014, one day before his 43rd birthday.

I returned to Sydney tired and sad, but I didn't realise the extent of my exhaustion until I spoke at a conference. At this supposed highlight of my career, I bolted offstage, powering on adrenaline, shaking and disoriented. When an acquaintance asked if I was okay and compassionately told me I looked awful, I realised I needed to stop. I spent days in bed feeling anxious, with a puffy face, aching muscles and a foggy brain. My doctor ordered tests and the results were bad. Most of my hormones were outside the healthy reference range.

I had to slow down and rebuild. I had to accept death and the chaos of life. I moderated my diet, alcohol intake and even

It's true... you can restore your healthy hormones with your fork. With the right nourishment, not only will your weight drop but your mind will be clear. If you find that you are hungry on this plan, you're doing something wrong.

noise exposure. I had to acknowledge that small achievements are enough. After this crash and with nothing left in the tank, I used food to heal. It took about twelve months to rebalance my hormones, and my thyroid is still adjusting, which is not uncommon following severe stress. I seek wellness for myself and for my family. And while I seek it, I've given up trying to live in an ivory tower. I'm not perfect.

Michele is always seeking evidence-based, high quality research to underpin her writing. As recognition of the good work they do, a percentage of the proceeds of the sale of this book will be donated to The Food & Mood Centre at Deakin University.

HOW TO USE THIS BOOK

PART 1 of this book is a quick introduction to hormones and how they can affect our weight, energy and mood.

PART 2 is a detailed examination of seven key hormones, accompanied by the stories of my clients who tackled and tamed them.

And **PART 3** is your day-by-day guide to the 28-day Hormone Rebalance: your ticket to hormone harmony and feeling like yourself again.

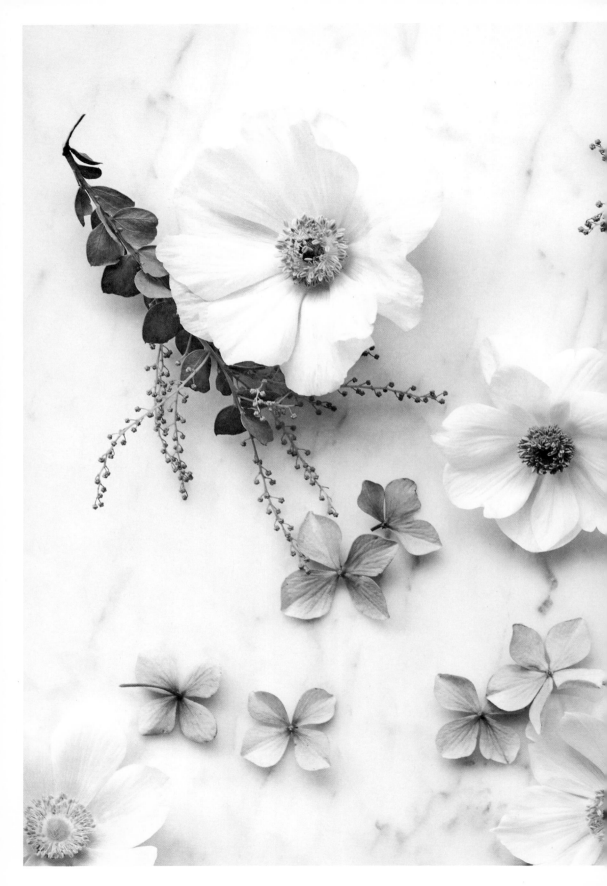

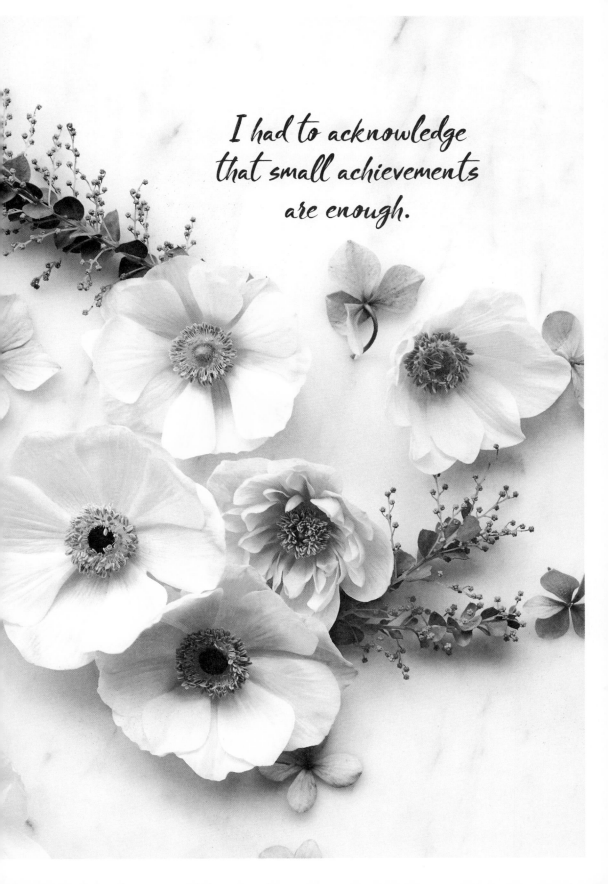

I had to acknowledge
that small achievements
are enough.

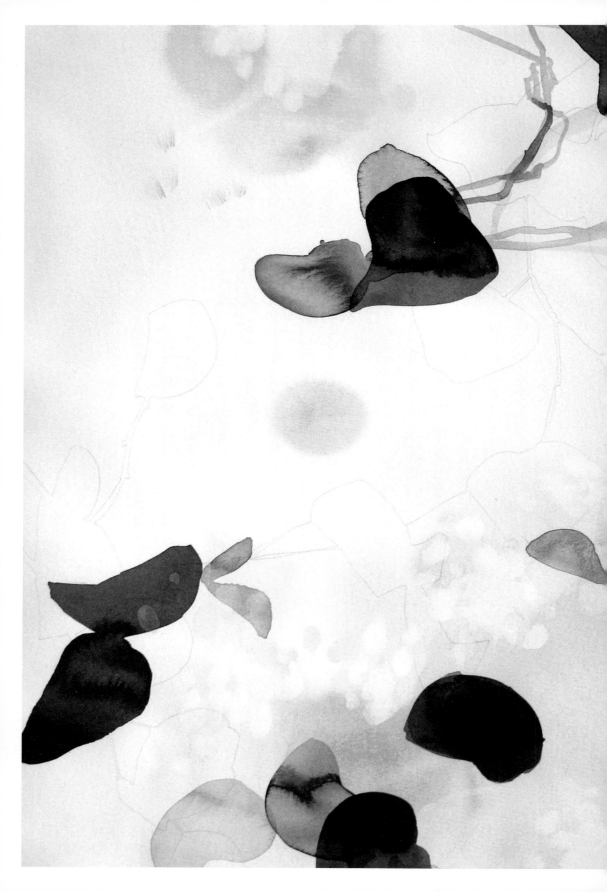

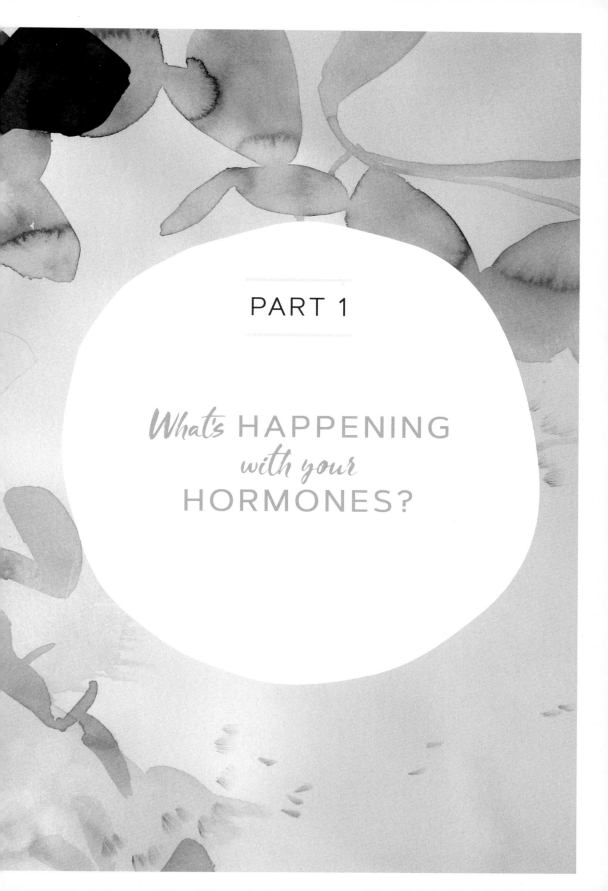

PART 1

What's HAPPENING with your HORMONES?

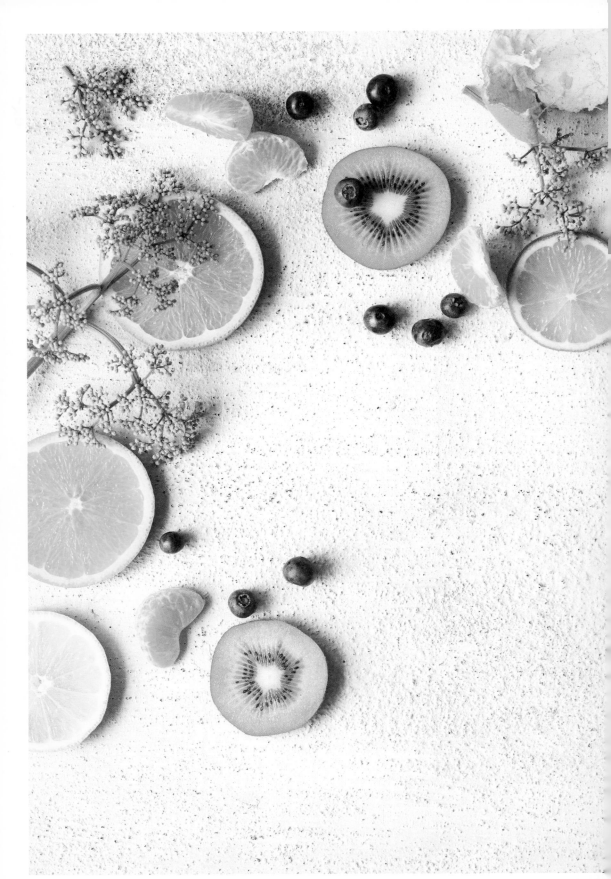

WHAT DO HORMONES DO?

Hormones control many bodily functions, including sleep, hunger, growth, mood and reproduction. Their ability to do this is affected by what we eat, how much sleep we get and our stress levels – no wonder they get out of whack.

When your brain receives a signal to send a specific hormone, that hormone is released from its source and travels through the bloodstream to its destination – the cell. It meets up with its matching hormone receptor and works its magic (a bit like searching for a friend in a crowded bar). That is unless the receptor or hormone is dysfunctional. Then the hormone can't do its job. Its levels rise or fall, affecting the behaviour of other hormones – and your weight, energy and mood.

Let me explain by describing a well-known hormone, insulin. Much of the food we eat breaks down into glucose, and the high levels of glucose in the bloodstream trigger the release of insulin into the bloodstream too. Insulin is the hormone that tells the cells to store the glucose for energy. If there's consistently too much glucose in the blood, over a period of time the insulin receptors on the cells close up shop and remove the slippery dips that bring glucose into the cells. You feel tired because glucose is no longer feeding your cells, and you also feel hungry because the cells are starved of fuel.

If the receptor becomes resistant in this way, glucose stays outside the cell (a bit like a kink in a hose that stops or slows the flow of water). This is what happens with insulin resistance. The cell becomes hungry for glucose, its source of nutrients and energy, but the insulin receptor has stopped responding. Glucose can't enter the cell and instead turns into tummy fat. Hello, muffin top. When our insulin receptors are dysfunctional, other hormones are likely to be affected too.

Hormones are the key to reclaiming your ideal weight, youthfulness and energy.

HORMONES AND WEIGHT

Hormones that affect weight, energy and mood (as shown opposite) include:

* **CORTISOL** *the stress hormone*
  Affects blood sugar levels, blood pressure and the immune system. When we feel stress, cortisol releases glucose. Too much cortisol causes fat to be stored on the belly.

* **INSULIN** *the fat-storage controller*
  Allows glucose entering cells to be used as energy. If there's too much glucose or the system is faulty, it's stored as fat. Chronically high insulin levels increase oestrogen and may lead to insulin resistance.

* **SEROTONIN** *the feel-good hormone*
  The mood stabiliser everyone wants to know more about. It affects our mood, appetite and sleep.

* **THYROID HORMONE** *the queen of metabolism*
  Affects metabolism, energy, sleep, weight and mood.

* **LEPTIN** *the hormone of hunger*
  Signals when we've had enough to eat. If it's not working properly, we do not receive the 'I am full and satiated' signal.

* **TESTOSTERONE** *the hormone of vitality*
  Affects energy, libido and lean muscle mass in men and women.

* **OESTROGEN** *the protective hormone*
  Produced in the ovaries, adrenal glands and fat cells. It affects brain function, the monthly cycle, skin elasticity, libido and mood.

In Part 2, you'll learn about each of these hormones in detail.

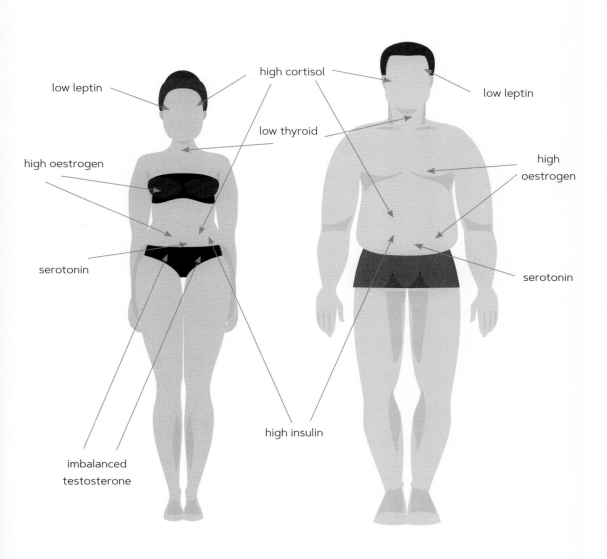

low leptin

high cortisol

low leptin

low thyroid

high oestrogen

high oestrogen

serotonin

serotonin

high insulin

imbalanced testosterone

WHAT CAUSES HORMONE CHAOS?

Hormone imbalances can strike at any age. But we often don't feel the full impact of hormone chaos until midlife. If you thrash yourself in your twenties and thirties, you pay for it when you reach your forties.

You know that demanding job you once had? You pushed yourself all day, went out drinking after work to relax and followed it up with a morning gym session before hitting repeat.

You weren't the only one working overtime – so were your adrenal glands. They responded to your pedal-to-the-metal lifestyle by sending out the adrenal hormones cortisol and adrenaline. Here's the clincher. Your body can handle toxic overload for many years before you see and feel the ramifications of too much alcohol, processed foods, excess calories, toxic cleaning products, sugars and prescription drugs. And then – BAM! You notice you don't bounce back from a big night out like you used to. And you just don't feel as good as you once did.

At my practice, I see a frightening number of younger women in hormone chaos, especially high achievers and go-getters. Their fast-paced lives mean they miss out on true nourishment. If their hormones could talk, these women would hear a lot from cortisol, which is released during stress. Eating grab-and-go foods puts them at risk of blood sugar dysregulation, insulin resistance and even polycystic ovarian

syndrome (PCOS), which affects fertility (see page 34).

It's likely this paced-up lifestyle features an invisible constant companion – stress. What happens during a typical day? The alarm jolts you awake. You race to the gym, grab a coffee after class, race back home, make sure the kids get off to school, feed the dog, deal with work, deadlines, office politics, pick up the kids, check in with other parents, prepare dinner, make sure the bills are paid, homework is done and extended family is okay, organise to catch up with friends, check Facebook. You collapse into bed but find it hard to wind down and sleep. And then you do it all again the next day. Leisure? That concept sounds so last century.

What's going on beneath the surface? Let's take a look at the effect of stress. On top of both kidneys are our tiny adrenal glands. Don't let their size fool you. They're vital to many bodily processes, including secreting cortisol and some of your oestrogen and testosterone. When an event occurs that our body registers as stressful, the adrenal glands release adrenaline, which increases our heart rate, blood pressure and carbohydrate metabolism, and slows our digestion. Then cortisol comes along with its friend glucose to provide energy for our muscles and brain. Back in our hunter-gatherer days, adrenaline and cortisol were released in response to an actual physical threat – in the form of, say, a sabre-toothed tiger – and this energy enabled us to run away. When we found a safe place, our cortisol levels returned to resting. But in our modern world, we have days, weeks and months of nonstop mild underlying stress generating a cascade of cortisol overload.

CORTISOL OVERLOAD HAS THESE CONSEQUENCES:

* It sends a signal that we must consume food to replace the fats and carbohydrates used during the real or perceived crisis. It stimulates our appetite and we feel ravenous. If stress is ongoing, our cortisol levels go up and stay up. This can cause us to 'stress-eat', because cortisol sends a signal that we're hungry. Just like a fuel symbol on a car dashboard, it pings at us to refuel our body.
* It contributes to insulin resistance. During times of chronic stress, our insulin levels go up and stay up. That's bad news for our waistline because of the link between stress, blood sugar and tummy fat.

Stress and cortisol can cancel out the benefits of healthy eating. In a study at Ohio State University, researchers tested markers of inflammation when women ate healthy and unhealthy types of fats. If the women had to deal with stressful events before eating their meal, the markers were worse, even if they had a meal made with healthier fats. The researchers believe it's the first study to show that stress has the potential to negate the benefits of healthy eating. Yikes!

I use the term 'slender ruster' to describe people who are outwardly slim but are suffering inflammation which causes oxidative damage, or 'rust', on the inside.

WHAT HAPPENS IF OUR HORMONES ARE UNBALANCED?

Since we're on the topic, let's crank up some more cortisol. Cortisol receives the fight-or-flight command and sends a message to glucose that extra energy is needed. You feel cravings and over time notice weight gain on your waist, because while glucose is stored in the liver, excess glucose is stored as fat. It also affects the levels of the calming hormone progesterone. But if your cortisol levels have been overloaded for too long, you can swing from high to low cortisol or adrenal exhaustion. You feel worn out. And we're only looking at the operation of one hormone. When you add oestrogen levels to the mix, too much can suppress the thyroid gland. If your thyroid is haywire, so are your mood and weight. If insulin is too high, it increases the risk of high testosterone that poses a risk for fertility and PCOS. The operation of hormones is intertwined.

It's common to blame a lack of willpower for poor eating decisions. But while this can be part of the equation, hormone hijackers also influence our eating decisions. It's not just cortisol sending signals to eat. Let me introduce you to the hormone that regulates hunger – leptin. When working well, it signals when we've eaten enough food. But if we develop leptin resistance, the signal isn't received and we feel hungry even when we've eaten enough to fuel our body's needs. It switches off and takes a holiday at our expense.

Our hormone levels can be affected by:

* training or overexercising
* stress and work commitments
* holidays and being in love
* eating well or badly
* shift work or poor sleep patterns
* the state of our liver
* allergies
* alcohol consumption.

Here's the good news. If you eat nutritious whole food, use practical techniques to de-stress, throw in some exercise and prioritise sleep, this can put you on the path to hormone harmony.

Hormonal imbalances felt as brain fog, cravings or low libido are often considered to be normal. Don't mistake common for normal.

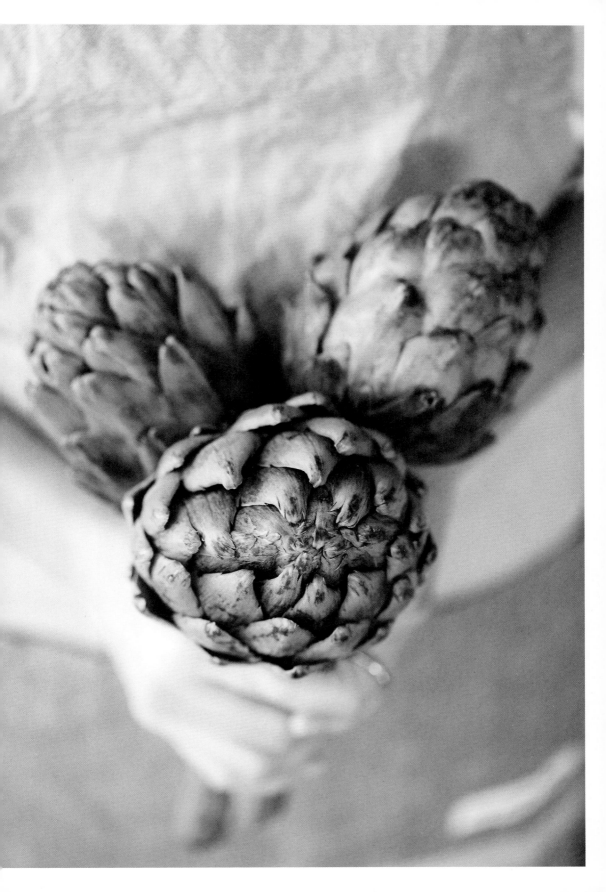

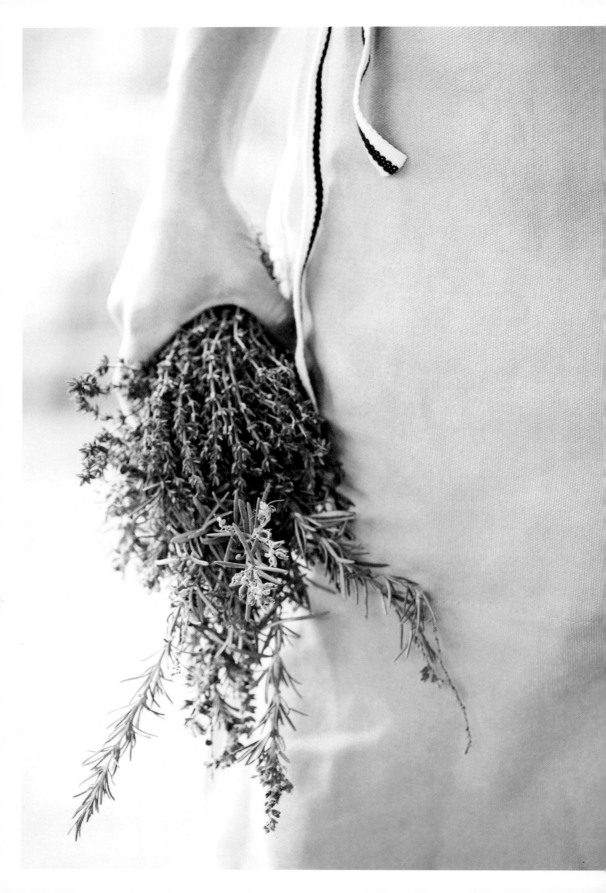

SHOULD YOU HAVE YOUR HORMONES TESTED?

I suggest a blood test every two years to find out what's going on inside your body and to check for signs of dysfunction. Of the seven hormones discussed in Part 2 of this book, only insulin and thyroid-stimulating hormone (TSH) are routinely tested. Hormones can be tricky to test. If a GP is looking for signs of perimenopause and menopause, they'll usually send you off for a hormone blood test. The GP can also test for oestrogen, progesterone, testosterone, dehydroepiandrosterone (DHEA) and cortisol levels. But the difficulty with hormone blood testing is that the levels change hourly, daily and monthly. Because everyone is different, there's no one-size-fits-all approach.

Apart from blood tests, there are two other ways to test hormone levels:

1 **Saliva hormone profiling** – performed by a practitioner in functional medicine, a qualified nutritionist or a naturopath. A saliva test can gauge sex hormones, DHEA and cortisol. These tests may be more expensive than blood tests.
2 **Hormone symptom profiling** – This is my preference. It's based on questionnaires, symptoms and listening to a client's history. The treatment involves nutrition and lifestyle modifications.

Whether you're experiencing weight gain, tiredness, low energy, mood swings or brain fog, following the 28-day Hormone Rebalance in Part 3 will improve your hormone levels, digestion, metabolism and mental function.

HRT AND THE 28-DAY HORMONE REBALANCE

Hormone replacement therapy (HRT) is taken by many women to lessen the effects of menopause. Doctors and specialists can advise you on the many options available. The 28-day Hormone Rebalance can be done in conjunction with taking HRT. I do believe, however, that good nutrition is the foundation for mental, physical and emotional health, and that no amount of medication or supplements can compensate for a poor diet. The rebalance is the perfect adjunct to modern medical approaches.

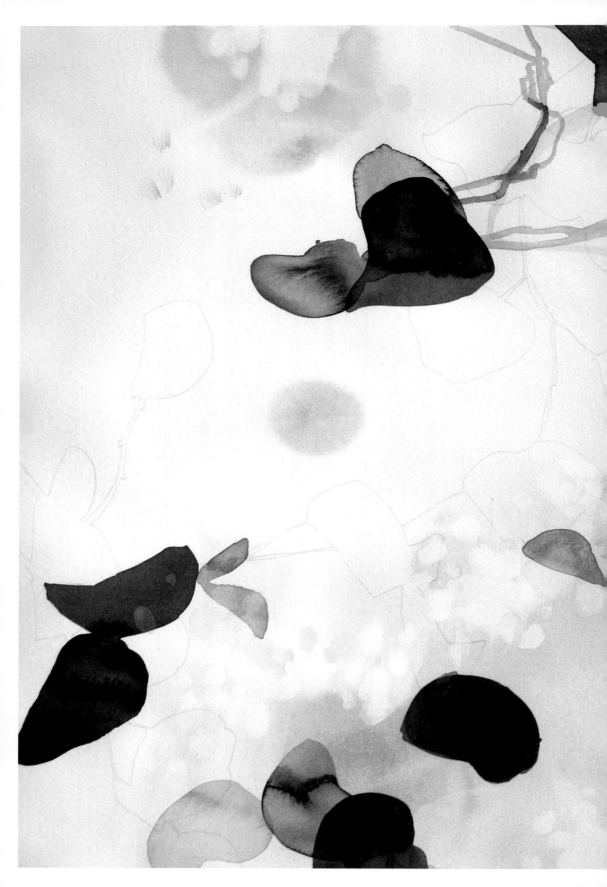

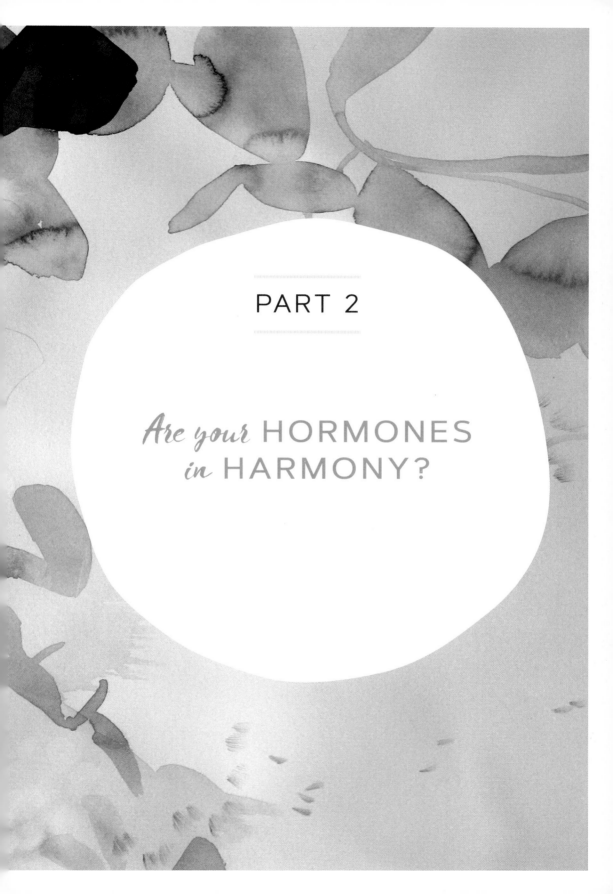

PART 2

Are your HORMONES in HARMONY?

ACHIEVING YOUR OWN
HORMONE HARMONY

In an ideal world, your hormones should behave like a gold-medal-winning Olympic synchronised swimming team. On cue, each should perform their designated role, creating a choreographed spectacle.

When our hormones are in sync, our energy levels resemble an evenly balanced seesaw and we feel good. This internal harmony is reflected in our appearance, from glowing skin to a lean body, bright eyes and shiny hair. But if our hormone levels are too high or too low, we feel it as low energy, irritability, sleep deprivation, brain fog or weight gain. It's as though one of our synchronised swimmers goes rogue and performs their own routine, creating a visual mess.

Computer science uses the phrase 'garbage in, garbage out' to describe what happens when poor-quality data is entered into a program. And the story is similar with diet and lifestyle. When we eat highly processed or low-nutrient food, our body doesn't get the best fuel. If we also add a busy family life, demanding career, financial pressures and lack of time, it's no wonder we're not firing on all cylinders. We're exhausted and unhappy with the way we look and feel. If you have issues with weight, energy, mood and libido, stop blaming yourself and your lack of willpower – let's look at your hormones.

In this section, you'll read the stories of my clients whose decision to deal with hormone chaos led to lifelong changes to their eating habits and lifestyle. And while each had different hormone imbalances, the solution was the same – ditching processed foods for quality whole foods, and finding ways to reduce stress and sleep well. A common theme was a high motivation to change. They had a trigger.

Most of us eat three to five times a day. This is effectively three to five opportunities to help our brain work more efficiently, our skin look clearer and our eyes brighter, and to improve our general wellbeing, so why not feed hunger and health at the same time? I call it nutritional transformation.

What does the happy and healthy version of you look like? Go ahead and write it down. Use this vision as motivation.

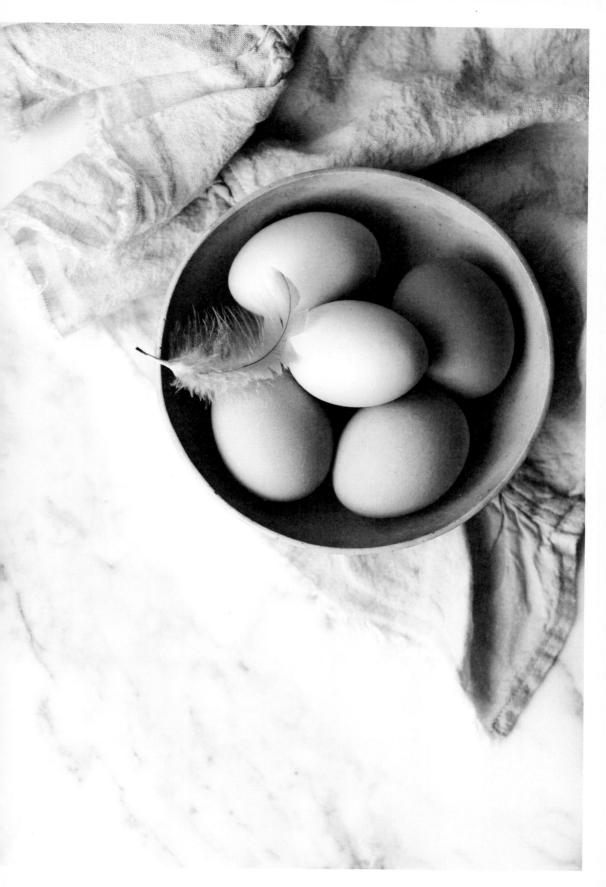

CORTISOL

the stress hormone

The adrenal glands, which are located at the top of the kidneys, produce the protective hormones cortisol, DHEA, adrenaline and noradrenaline. They operate in the same way as shock absorbers in a car and help us bounce back from everyday stress. When we face a real or perceived stressor, these hormones allow glucose to be released from cells to power the heart and muscles to take action. In hunter-gatherer times, it meant running away from danger.

Today, in the absence of physical danger, the body pumps out cortisol and glucose to power the muscles and help us run away to safety, but there is no running away, and that extra energy is felt as restlessness or irritability. Excessively high levels of adrenaline caused by stress may cause a nervous feeling, glucose overload, insomnia and heart damage. They decrease levels of the happy hormone, serotonin, and increase levels of cholesterol and fats in the blood.

Healthy, balanced levels of cortisol help control blood sugar levels and blood pressure, regulate metabolism, reduce inflammation and ensure memory formation. In women, cortisol also supports the developing fetus during pregnancy. Many women today have an imbalance of cortisol – either too much or too little.

DO YOU HAVE A CORTISOL IMBALANCE?

* Do you have low energy during the day but feel wired at night?
* Do you feel as though you're constantly racing from one task to the next, even if the racing is only in your head?
* Do you find it difficult to feel calm even in a yoga or meditation class?
* Are you very emotional?
* Do you feel forgetful?
* Do you crave sweet foods?
* Do you use caffeine to perk yourself up during the day and use wine to soothe your nerves in the evening?
* Do you have a 'muffin top', 'love handles' or 'Betty back fat'?
* Do you have low bone density or osteoporosis?
* Do you have insulin or blood-sugar issues?
* Do you have painful periods?

If you answered yes to three or more of these questions, you could have a cortisol imbalance. Consult your GP, qualified nutritionist or other health professional for the go-ahead to follow the 28-day Hormone Rebalance. If your symptoms persist, you may need further medical assistance.

HOW TO REBALANCE CORTISOL

1. Eat more, but eat better

Most people are incredibly apprehensive when I tell them to eat more. But it's about changing the *type* of food they eat – the nutrient quality. Think about this. It's easy to eat five Tim Tams in one go, but not so easy to eat five avocados. And soon after eating the Tim Tams, you're hungry again. The difference is nutrient quality. Food eaten during the rebalance sends a signal to the brain that says: 'Hey, I feel quite content. I don't need to keep eating.'

2. Sleep more

If you don't sleep well, you're more likely to gain weight. In a long-term study in the United States called the Nurses' Health Study, women who slept for fewer than five hours a night were 2.4 kilograms heavier than those who slept for seven hours a night. When we're tired, we feel grumpy, and are more likely to eat poorly and less motivated to exercise. Sleep is important for weight stabilisation, and its restorative effects can be seen in our skin and eyes and felt in our thoughts and mood. Lack of sleep contributes to insulin resistance, leptin resistance, obesity, carbohydrate cravings, depression, hormone dysfunction and accelerated ageing.

3. Cut out the booze

Here's the thing with alcohol: it does initially allow us to feel relaxed, but it's what happens when we go to sleep that's the problem. Yes, we sleep more deeply at first, but as the alcohol dissipates in our system, we tend to come out of deep sleep and into REM sleep, which is easier to wake from. That's why we often wake up after a few hours. During the night, we have six or seven cycles of REM sleep, but if we've been drinking, we only have about one or two. Translation: we feel exhausted. Alcohol also inhibits the operation of the parasympathetic nervous system – our 'rest and digest' system – reducing the restorative function of sleep. And alcohol depletes B vitamins – the vitamins of energy. Vitamin B6 and an amino acid called tryptophan are necessary to make the feel-good hormone, serotonin.

During the rebalance, you should cut out alcohol completely. Some of you will follow this strictly but others will find it impossible not to indulge. If you must, only allow yourself two drinks a week and not on the same night. After you've completed the rebalance and found renewed energy, I hope you'll take a modest approach to drinking – one or two standard-sized drinks in a sitting with several alcohol-free nights each week. And remember, standard-sized means 100 ml rather than a free pour. Once your body feels a sense of balance, control and health, you may not want to overindulge or binge on alcohol or food.

4. Exercise moderately

Even though it doesn't feel like it at the time, our bodies love to work up a sweat. When we exercise, it lowers our blood glucose levels and increases insulin sensitivity. This means the cells can use insulin to take up glucose during and after exercise. Exercise, particularly high-intensity interval training (HIIT) and strength training, increases metabolism or the rate at which the body burns calories for energy. It also helps increase lean body mass – weight minus fat. The more muscle we have, the better. But here's the dilemma. When we thrash ourselves during exercise, it can become another form of stress that can hinder weight loss. You therefore need to find a balance. Rather than 'extreme exercise' all the time, incorporate low-stress movement in your day such as walking, yoga or Pilates. Consider the impact your activity will have on your cortisol levels. Don't get me wrong – an intense workout and endorphin release can make you feel fantastic, but not if it's on top of other stress.

5. Reduce stress

Regardless of what causes us to feel stressed – from financial worries to eating sugary foods – the impact on our body is the same. One trigger for cortisol release is a busy, stressful routine. The alarm bursts you from a morning dream, you jump into action, drink a coffee, get the kids off to school, feed the dog, do a load of washing, tidy up, go to the gym, get to work, pretend you're calm, go home, cook dinner, wash up, be a good parent, then go to bed tired but wired.

Chronic or ongoing stress leads to consistently elevated levels of glucose, increased blood sugar and eventually insulin resistance. Over time, it means glucose can't cross into our cells to provide energy, and we feel tired and hungry. It can lead to insulin resistance, prediabetes or metabolic syndrome – three similar health conditions that all lead to type 2 diabetes. The excess glucose is stored as belly fat or, in extreme cases, a cortisol or 'buffalo' hump behind the shoulders. When we're stressed, we're more likely to eat comfort food to feel better.

Are you someone who loses weight when on holiday? If so, take time to work out how your stressful life is contributing to your love handles. In addition, your body doesn't differentiate between the stress generated from a frantic life and the stress caused by poor food choices. As far as your body is concerned, it's just stress. It has the same biochemical reaction – in particular, cortisol release. When you learn to deal with stress, you won't have as much cortisol swirling around in your system.

Become aware of when you feel the effects of stress. Notice when you feel rushed or overwhelmed. Catch yourself and pause. Breathe. Take it one task at a time. When you feel stressed, tap into your senses – what can you see, hear, feel, taste and touch? Seek out alternative methods to lower stress such as meditation, yoga, walking or just talking with a friend.

Are you someone who loses weight when on holiday? If so, take time to work out how your stressful life is contributing to your love handles.

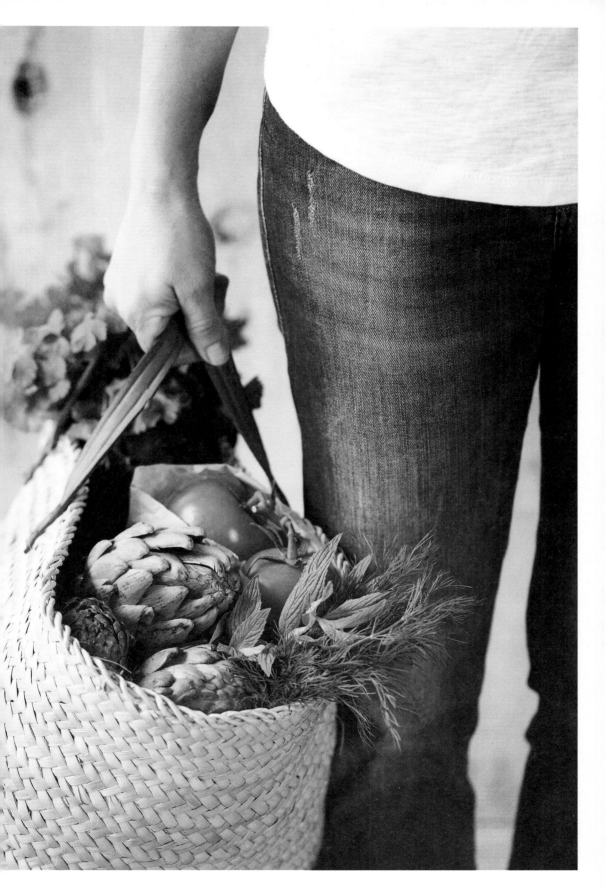

BARBARA'S HIGHWIRE LIFESTYLE

When Barbara looked through some family photos taken on a recent holiday, she felt a jolt. Despite the idyllic beach setting, all she could see were her stomach and what she describes as a generous muffin top spilling over her shorts.

She was 48 years old, married with two teenage sons and working full time as an accountant. During an appointment at my clinic, she told me she was fed up with always feeling tired and thought she might have chronic fatigue syndrome, a thyroid problem or the beginnings of menopause.

Barbara said her weight was normal until she had children. From that time, she carried an additional 6–8 kilograms that she couldn't shift, even though she exercised regularly and often starved herself. The more she exercised and starved, the more weight she seemed to gain. Barbara was also motivated to do something about her weight because her perimenopausal friends had warned her about weight gain when menopause came along.

When I asked Barbara about her eating patterns, she said she ate 'like a bird' during the day, but for dinner she usually consumed more food than she should. She often drank two to three glasses of wine to wind down from her hectic day and would generally 'hunt down' some chocolate. When she went to bed, she felt exhausted but wired and she didn't sleep as soundly as she used to. When

her alarm went off at 6 am, she awoke annoyed with herself for overeating at dinner and for the chocolate-eating frenzy, and headed to the gym. She loved taking the cycle class because it was loud and fast, and she pushed herself to burn off the calories 'inhaled' the previous night. After the gym, she raced to work.

Barbara's workday was filled with client meetings and regular deadlines. Her colleagues probably thought she had everything under control, but in her mind she raced from one task to the next. She was like a duck treading water – calm on the surface but with her feet constantly moving beneath. Because she was so busy during the day, she didn't plan her meals and often grabbed a muffin and double-shot latte for breakfast. On some days it was two lattes. Lunch was a salad sandwich or smoothie and another double-shot latte. And she didn't eat again until dinner. When I asked her if she felt hungry at around 3 pm, she quipped, 'Oh yes. But it's more like hangry – hungry and angry.' In the afternoon, she drank a cup of tea and snacked on a handful of naturally flavoured and coloured snakes or jelly babies in the belief that they were a healthier choice. Dinner was often based around pasta because it was easy to make and her sons liked it.

Even though she went to bed at the reasonable time of 10 pm, Barbara only slept for around six hours. Lying in bed, she was in the habit of checking Facebook and responding to texts sent to her during the day. This made her feel wired instead of tired. Before she knew it, it was almost midnight when she actually went to sleep.

Barbara's cortisol levels were three times the recommended level. I'd suspected as much after hearing the descriptions of her demanding career, extreme gym workouts and poor sleep patterns. I asked her if she lost weight when on holidays and she said she did. This is very common for people with cortisol overload – when their body is calm, they unintentionally lose weight. She didn't use relaxation techniques and her poor nutrition choices caused her blood sugar levels to rise and become deposited as belly fat. Barbara's high cortisol levels caused insulin resistance that put pressure on her thyroid hormones because changes in one hormone create a cascading effect. Barbara's blood tests also revealed she was prediabetic. Having watched her mother and aunt become type 2 diabetics in their mid-fifties, she was motivated to make some changes.

My advice to Barbara

My surprising advice to Barbara was to eat more food. But there was a catch. She needed to cut out processed foods and increase her intake of high-quality protein such as fish, grass-fed beef and free-range chicken, and of high-quality fats. Barbara also admitted to a 'generous pour' when serving wine, which meant she drank more than the standard 100 ml drink size.

I advised her to cut out alcohol during the rebalance.

I also told Barbara that the exercise she was doing was counterproductive: she participated in 'stationary bike rage'. After a frantic race to the gym, there was another race to secure a bike for the cycle class followed by 45 minutes of loud music and profuse sweating. This only served to increase her cortisol levels and prevent weight loss.

Barbara's results

Barbara balanced her calorie intake across the day by eating three meals and two protein-based snacks. Because she wasn't hungry, she didn't eat whatever food came across her path in the evening, and she didn't need a big dinner because she was well nourished. She also worked on winding down before going to bed, and she banned her phone from the bedroom. She said this helped with her energy and concentration during the day. At 3 pm, when she used to have a midafternoon slump and reach for lollies, she now grabs a handful of nuts to eat with her cup of tea.

After twelve weeks, Barbara's blood tests showed normal fasting insulin, glucose levels and cortisol levels. Her LDL (bad) cholesterol level dropped from 3.6 to 3.3. When she stepped on the scales measuring body composition, they revealed a reduction in weight, increase in muscle mass and greater cellular hydration. She said, 'I like what I see in the mirror. It's the younger me: calm, lean and healthy-looking.'

INSULIN
the fat-storage controller

Insulin is made in the pancreas and allows the body to use carbohydrates for energy, unless it fails to operate. Insulin is often the key to weight issues. It can become off-balance for a number of reasons and, once it's out of whack, it's very difficult to lose weight.

When we eat certain foods, they break down into a simple form of sugar called glucose. Glucose in the bloodstream triggers the pancreas to release insulin, the hormone that tells the cells to store this glucose for energy. If there's consistently too much glucose and thus too much insulin, the insulin receptors on the cells cease to react, and no longer take up the glucose. This is often the start of insulin resistance or prediabetes. It leads to tiredness because glucose is no longer feeding the cell, and to hunger because the cell is starved of fuel (glucose).

When there's excess insulin, a message is sent to the brain about another hormone, leptin. Leptin is the hormone that sends a signal to the brain to say, 'Thank you for that food. I'm full and satisfied. I'll stop the hunger thoughts now.' But too much insulin can block the leptin signal in the brain and cause leptin resistance. So even though you've had enough to eat, your brain still sends a signal that you're hungry (for more about leptin see page 56).

You may not realise the amount of sugar you're consuming because packaged foods and alcohol often contain hidden sugars. These cause excess insulin to be released, and over time insulin resistance develops. When insulin levels spike after eating a meal high in sugar, levels of a substance called sex hormone binding globulin (SHBG) can drop, which is a problem because SHBG binds to excess oestrogen in the blood. You want SHBG to be balanced in order to remove rather than recirculate excess oestrogen. It's that cascade effect again – the behaviour of one hormone impacts the behaviour of another. You'll find out soon why you don't want excess oestrogen (see page 62).

Insulin is also implicated in polycystic ovarian syndrome (PCOS). PCOS has many causes, including genetics, lifestyle, chronic stress and toxic exposure. The current epidemic of PCOS is largely fuelled by blood sugar dysregulation. Women with PCOS may have high insulin levels, which create unwanted testosterone. The heartbreak is the number of women who are unaware that blood sugar dysregulation and PCOS are so closely tied. At the time of writing, there was a proposal to rename PCOS 'metabolic reproductive syndrome', to reflect the complex nature of the condition. Many women don't know that nutrition and lifestyle changes can assist with fertility.

DO YOU HAVE AN INSULIN IMBALANCE?

* Do you crave sweet foods? When you eat sweet foods, do you feel good initially, but then your mood drops?
* Do you have a family history of type 2 diabetes?
* Do you get the shakes 2–3 hours after eating?
* Do you find it hard to lose weight?
* Do you get cranky/tired if you miss a meal?
* If you eat processed carbs at breakfast, such as toast or cereal, do you find it hard to control what you eat during the day?
* Do you feel good if you eat fish, meat or veggies?
* Do you feel like your energy levels fall after eating bread, pasta or potatoes?
* Are you prone to fungal infections (thrush, scaly patches on the skin)?
* Do you suffer from mood swings?

If you answered yes to three or more of these questions, you could have an insulin imbalance. Consult your GP, qualified nutritionist or other health professional for the go-ahead to follow the 28-day Hormone Rebalance. If your symptoms persist, you may need further medical assistance.

HOW TO REBALANCE INSULIN

1. Eat well

Fill your fridge and pantry with healthy and satisfying food (see page 80). Increase the amount of protein and fat in every meal, which will make you less likely to grab a sugary snack during the mid-afternoon slump that will cause a blood sugar spike.

2. De-stress

Stress is a risk factor for polycystic ovary syndrome (PCOS), among other things. As we've seen, when we feel stress, our body's fight-or-flight response kicks in. The adrenal glands and brain release adrenaline, cortisol and noradrenaline. These messengers increase blood flow to the heart, lungs, muscles and brain to help us fight or run away. Cortisol increases in the amount of glucose in the blood to provide energy for muscles. This is fantastic if stress is short-lived, but these days stress is constant – both underlying and overt. Increased glucose in the bloodstream may lead to insulin resistance, one of the main culprits in PCOS.

3. Sleep well

If your sleep is poor, it adds fuel to the PCOS fire. In one study, overall insulin sensitivity was 16 per cent lower after four nights of sleep deprivation compared to a normal night of sleep. The sensitivity of fat cells to insulin dropped by 30 per cent, to levels typically seen in people who are obese or have type 2 diabetes. According to the lead researcher, Professor Matthew Brady of the University of Chicago, 'This is the equivalent of metabolically aging someone ten to twenty years just from four nights of partial sleep restriction. Fat cells need sleep, and when they don't get enough sleep, they become metabolically groggy.' This is only one of many studies that underline the importance of sleep for health.

STRESSED STEPHANIE SEEMS HEALTHY

Stephanie is always punctual. Working at an advertising agency as a creative director, she's often the first to arrive at the office. The job is demanding, but she enjoys pushing projects to the finishing line and is a self-described A-type personality.

Steph thought that becoming pregnant would be relatively straightforward. She was 30 years old and healthy. But after six unsuccessful months, she saw a specialist who diagnosed PCOS and post-pill amenorrhea (a loss of periods from taking birth-control pills). 'I was advised that my hormone imbalances and type-A stress levels were preventing me from having a natural cycle,' Steph told me, 'and that my chances of ever falling pregnant were next to nothing. For someone who always wanted a family, you can imagine how devastated I was.' I reassured Steph that PCOS has many causes, but in her case, diet could be the culprit.

Steph was slim and ate whatever she wanted. Breakfast was a bowl of cereal, morning tea a banana muffin and lunch was usually pasta. For afternoon tea, she'd drink a smoothie. Her go-to dinner was Thai takeaway. She was a true grab-and-go eater, choosing food she could consume quickly. Her meals lacked quality fats, protein and slow-burning carbs.

She often found it hard to get to sleep as the events of the day swirled around in her head. I see tired-but-wired clients every day and recognised these patterns from my own time in the corporate sector – including Steph's desire to please everyone and climb the corporate ladder. And there's nothing wrong with these aspirations, as long as you don't dismiss your health along the way.

Like many women, Steph thought her diet was healthy. I remember her shock when I outlined the extent of hidden sugars and unhealthy fats in the processed and packaged foods in her pantry. The muffin had 10 teaspoons of sugar and the 'healthy' smoothie had 22 teaspoons of sugar! Many were labelled 'healthy', 'natural' and 'gluten-free'. When we uncovered that Steph was consuming 40–44 teaspoons of sugar a day, she was angry with herself and outraged that there was so much hidden sugar in so-called healthy foods. A stressful job contributed to her grab-and-go food choices and poor sleep patterns – another risk factor in insulin resistance. Steph had many hormones firing and misfiring. In particular, her insulin levels were causing high testosterone – a sign of PCOS. She had to make improvements to her nutrition and reduce her stress levels.

And she's not alone. Many young professional women are chronically stressed and at risk of adrenal fatigue, chronic fatigue, fertility issues and autoimmune diseases. There is also concern about a link between stress and breast cancer.

My advice to Steph

I began with the concept of 'crowding in' healthy, satisfying foods, so that Steph wouldn't be tempted to turn to junk foods. I then advised her to increase her intake of good-quality proteins and fats. She also badly needed to improve her sleep patterns and find a means of reducing her stress.

Steph's results

After the rebalance, Steph was tested again: 'The results were the same. I was advised that I wouldn't fall pregnant because there was no evidence of a natural cycle.' Despite this setback, she and her husband carried on with their new nutrition plan and lifestyle. 'One day my husband said, "I think you're pregnant." The next week at a function a girlfriend commented on how "full" I looked in my dress. It was only when I returned home from a work trip and was ill that I decided to take a test. After three or four tests, all positive, I was in absolute delightful shock and drove straight to the clinic for a blood test, which confirmed I was 9 weeks pregnant. I felt a combination of happiness and puzzlement. The clinic said it was "spontaneous ovulation", but I knew otherwise. I still eat really well and keep an eye on my friend and foe – sugar. I have a 16-month-old toddler and another child on the way. I'm so pleased I stopped to take care of myself and bring the most joy and happiness into my life – a miracle family.'

THE DANGERS OF A 'SLENDER RUSTER'

Early in my first consultation with Steph, I identified her as a 'slender ruster' – someone who is outwardly slim but whose internal system is inflamed from oxidative stress. Steph was 'rusting' on the inside. The results of her blood tests revealed a fasting insulin level three times higher than normal, and abnormal testosterone levels. When she described her lifestyle, I suspected she had elevated cortisol levels, because she was either 100 per cent on or completely off – there was no happy medium. She believed relaxation was a waste of productive time.

Those diagnosed with metabolic syndrome suffer greater levels of oxidative stress than healthier people. Oxidative stress occurs when there are more damaging free radicals than healthy antioxidants. Sugar consumption is also implicated in premature skin ageing because sugar increases oxidative stress and destroys elastin and collagen in a process called advanced glycation end-products (also known as AGEs, rather ironically!).

THYROID
the queen of metabolism

The thyroid, a small butterfly-shaped gland in the throat, is the queen of metabolism, producing the master metabolism hormones. Thyroid hormones interact with insulin, cortisol, oestrogen and testosterone, but the thyroid trumps these hormones. If your thyroid is out of kilter, so are your mood, energy, weight and brain clarity.

One in four female patients at my clinic has a subclinical thyroid. The term 'subclinical' means the body is waving a warning flag saying, 'Help! I'm struggling.' But even with this warning flag, a blood test may not reveal full-blown thyroid disease. When thyroid-stimulating hormone (TSH) levels are too low, this may indicate hyperthyroidism. If they're too high, it may be hypothyroidism. (Just the opposite of what you might assume!)

Low thyroid function is common in women. More than 70 per cent of those with thyroid problems have a family history of thyroid dysfunction. It can also be caused by exposure to toxins or viruses, giving birth (postpartum thyroiditis), autoimmune diseases (Graves' disease or Hashimoto's disease), stress and age. One endocrinologist told me it's only in the last twenty years that GPs have consistently tested the thyroid when patients complain of low energy and mood. Before this, women were often

thought to be depressed or going through early menopause.

The usual test for thyroid issues is a blood test for thyroid-stimulating hormone (TSH). But TSH doesn't paint the entire thyroid picture. Thyroid antibodies are important factors, as are T3 (triiodothyronine) and T4 (thyroxine). T3 and T4 are the hormones that actually deliver the thyroid messages to cells, with a key stop at the liver to convert inactive T4 into active T3 followed by a message to regulate metabolism and cholesterol levels. Our thyroid makes prednisolone from cholesterol, which is further refined into progesterone, the calming hormone. This delicate interplay can be upset by poor diet, infection and stress. In addition, there's a process that produces what is called reverse T3 (RT3), a metabolite of T4. In some cases the body conserves energy by converting T4 into RT3, an inactive form of T3 incapable of delivering oxygen and energy to cells.

If you have symptoms of depression, hair loss, fatigue, muscle pain, sensitivity to cold and heat, fluid retention or constipation, in addition to checking TSH levels, I recommend that you ask for a test of thyroid antibodies and free T3 and T4, even if it means paying extra money for the test to be taken.

In some cases, thyroid sluggishness can be restored and underpinned by nutritional and lifestyle support, but it often requires the intervention of an endocrinologist if medication is also required. Eating foods high in nutrients and antioxidants can, however, support you significantly if you have thyroid dysfunction.

WHAT CAUSES THYROID DYSFUNCTION?

Common causes of thyroid issues include:

* **autoimmune diseases** – In these, the immune system attacks the thyroid gland. Graves' disease and Hashimoto's are the diagnoses when there is an autoimmune component. It can be triggered by a number of factors, including genetics, toxic exposure to mercury or other environmental toxins, a deficiency of vitamin D or other nutrients, and gluten intolerance.
* **selenium deficiency** – Modern farming

techniques mean our vegetables are often deficient in the immune-building mineral selenium, which is necessary to create active thyroid hormone (see page 41).

* **excess oestrogen** – Too much of this powerful hormone (see page 62) can suppress thyroid function.
* **environmental toxins** – Bisphenol A (BPA) and polychlorinated biphenyl (PCB), which are still used in some plastic water bottles and takeaway food containers, can leach toxins into foods.
* **too much stress** – Cortisol levels can interfere with thyroid-stimulating hormone (TSH). Stress is one of the environmental triggers for thyroid issues.
* **low iodine** – A fine balance of iodine is necessary for proper thyroid function, and breast and brain health. Too much or too little iodine can worsen conditions.

FACTORS THAT **AFFECT THYROID FUNCTION**

T4 (inactive)

T3 (active)

cell

Factors that contribute to proper production of thyroid hormones

* Nutrients: iron, iodine, tyrosine, zinc, selenium, vitamin E, B2, B3, B6, C, D

Factors that inhibit proper production of thyroid hormones

* Stress
* Infection, trauma, radiation, medications
* Fluoride (antagonist to iodine)
* Toxins: pesticides, mercury, cadmium, lead
* Autoimmune disease: coeliac

Factors that improve cellular sensitivity to thyroid hormones

* Vitamin A
* Exercise
* Selenium
* Zinc

DO YOU HAVE A THYROID IMBALANCE?

* Do you have a family history of thyroid issues?
* Do you feel tired after exercise, in the afternoon or throughout the day?
* Do you have unexplained swelling?
* Do you find it hard to get out of bed even after eight or nine hours of sleep?
* Do you feel the cold more quickly than other people?
* Are your hands and feet often the first to feel the cold?
* Do you suffer from constipation?
* Is the final quarter of your eyebrow missing or wispy?
* Do you crave sugary foods?
* When you miss a meal, do you feel shaky?
* Is your skin dry and itchy?
* Do you find it hard to lose weight?
* Do you sweat only a little?
* Do you have brain fog, or memory or concentration issues?
* Do you often feel depressed, moody or irritable?
* Do you have low libido?
* Do you look puffy or bloated, especially around the eyes?
* Do you need a lot of sleep?
* Do you have low blood pressure?

If you answered yes to eight or more of these questions, you could have a thyroid imbalance. Most people have low rather than high levels of thyroid hormone. Consult your GP, qualified nutritionist or other health professional for the go-ahead to follow the 28-day Hormone Rebalance. If your symptoms persist, you may need further medical assistance.

SYMPTOMS OF THYROID IMBALANCE

An underactive thyroid gland or Hashimoto's disease can lead to:

* depression and exhaustion (despite a good night's sleep)
* difficulty losing weight
* dry and puffy-looking skin
* memory problems
* loss of hair
* loss of the outer quarter of the eyebrows
* slow bowels
* sensitivity to cold.

An overactive thyroid or Graves' disease can lead to:

* weakness and weight loss
* nervousness
* heat intolerance
* fast heartbeat (tachycardia)
* loose stools.

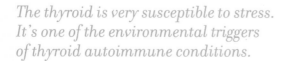

The thyroid is very susceptible to stress. It's one of the environmental triggers of thyroid autoimmune conditions.

WHY TEST FOR MORE THAN TSH?

The ideal range for TSH is 1–2 mIU/ml. According to leading functional medical practitioner Dr Mark Hyman, the diagnosis of subclinical hypothyroidism (with mild or no symptoms) depends on a TSH level of 5–10 mIU/ml, while new guidelines suggest that anything over 3 mIU/ml is abnormal. While these guidelines are an improvement, practitioners using them could still miss someone who has normal TSH test results but a malfunctioning thyroid. This is why I recommend also testing free T3 and T4 thyroid antibodies.

HOW TO REBALANCE THYROID HORMONE

The 28-day Hormone Rebalance is about creating a 'clean slate'. The process is similar to an elimination diet, but I prefer to describe it as a clean slate because it's about filling your plate with so much good food it doesn't feel like elimination. It removes those foods that can cause irritation, sensitivities or full-blown allergies. When inflammatory foods such as gluten and dairy are removed, many people experience immediate and positive results.

1. Cut out gluten

If you have a thyroid issue, either high or low, I suggest removing gluten and dairy from your diet because both can be inflammatory. When we eat gluten, or foods that are irritating but not necessarily allergenic, it can cause what's known as leaky gut. This occurs when the lining of the gut develops tiny gaps between the cells that make up the membrane wall. It becomes irritated by foods to which we are sensitive or allergic. Rather than absorb nutrients as it should, the holes allow toxins, microbes and undigested food to sneak from the digestive tract into the bloodstream, where the body interprets them as invaders. It creates an immune response, which often manifests as something unpleasant, such as puffiness, nervousness, sleeplessness and numerous other subtle health hijackers. It attacks organs associated with the thyroid or digestive systems, which then don't operate as well as they should.

If you miss your bread fix, try gluten-free bread made from buckwheat. While it has 'wheat' in its name, buckwheat is a pseudo-cereal made from a non-gluten grain. I recommend it over other non-gluten and rice bread because it's low-carb and very high in nutrients.

2. Increase your intake of mineral-rich foods

The thyroid requires the right levels of minerals to function well. We used to obtain these trace minerals from foods grown in soil, but changes in farming techniques mean that these levels are often too low. Foods high in selenium, which assist thyroid function, include tuna, sardines, prawns, mushrooms, yoghurt and spinach. Eat a small handful of selenium-rich brazil nuts in the morning or afternoon every other day.

Iodine is essential for brain health, metabolism and the thyroid. Before taking an iodine supplement or eating high-iodine foods, consult a nutritionist or your GP, because too much iodine can be as detrimental to health as too little. Good sources of iodine include Himalayan salt, dulse flakes (added to salads, soups and casseroles), yoghurt, eggs, tuna, butter beans, corn, prunes, and dried edible seaweed such as kelp.

Despite cutting out gluten, don't be carb-phobic – eating too few carbohydrates can affect your thyroid. But when you eat a carb food such as gluten-free oats, halve the serving of oats and add a little protein food, such as seeds and yoghurt. The protein will balance your blood sugar levels and good fats, keeping you feeling full. Or toast one slice of buckwheat bread and pile it high with guacamole rather than eating two slices of buckwheat bread.

If you have hypothyroidism, there are specific dietary recommendations to follow:

* **Avoid raw cruciferous vegetables** – Uncooked cabbage, brussels sprouts, broccoli, broccolini, bok choy, cauliflower, turnip, watercress and kale contain isothiocyanates, which appear to block some thyroid functions. These are some of my favourite foods, especially for cleansing the liver. Luckily, you can eliminate the effect on the thyroid gland by cooking them. Even mild heat alters their molecular structure – sautéed, slightly blanched or barbecued will do.
* **Avoid non-fermented soy** – Soy phytoestrogens are not good for the thyroid. Remove soy milk, tofu and soy cheese from your shopping list. You can replace them with fermented soy products, such as miso and tempeh.
* **Avoid bromine** – Bromine is an endocrine disruptor and interferes with the absorption of iodine by the thyroid gland. It can be found in bread, baked goods, soft drinks and sports drinks.

3. Turn off the chaos and de-stress

The thyroid is very susceptible to stress. It's one of the environmental triggers of thyroid autoimmune conditions. Even though most thyroid problems are attributable to genetics, environmental factors can also play a role in susceptible individuals. These environmental factors include infections, stress, iodine intake, smoking, medications such as amiodarone (for abnormal heart rhythms) and interferon (for cancer), radiation and environmental toxins such as triclosan (an antibacterial compound in many soaps) and BPAs (in plastics).

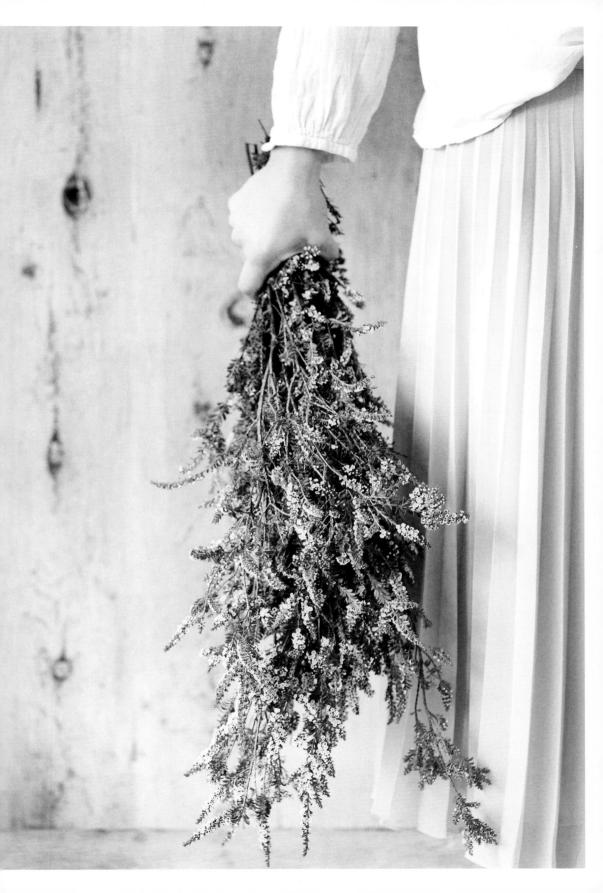

LUCIA IS LAID LOW

Before becoming a mum to two girls, Lucia, now aged 40, worked as a financial trader, spending twelve years in a competitive and adrenaline-fuelled environment. She then established an importing business before scaling back her responsibilities because of issues with her health. During Lucia's first consultation with me, she complained about gaining weight. She was particularly frustrated and perplexed because she hadn't changed her diet.

As we continued chatting, she said she was really tired, her joints felt achy and her brain was muddled. 'I'm really nervous that I have the beginnings of dementia,' she shared. 'It feels as though my once-sharp memory has run away.' She said it was difficult to focus on reading a book or newspaper. Lucia had noticed these changes following the birth of her second child four years earlier. It was around this time she sold part of her share of the business to her partner because she lacked energy and concentration. Lucia said, 'I feel puffy. My face is puffy and I feel bloated.' She said her bowel movements had slowed to twice a week and her poo was like pebbles. Her periods had gone from being like clockwork to happening any time from 35 to 45 days apart, if at all, and they were sometimes very heavy. Because of her achy joints, Lucia had scaled back her exercise. 'I feel as though I'm in a cycle of feeling tired, eating to get energy and being scared there's something's wrong with my memory. I'm a shadow of my former self.' She remembered a time when she felt vibrant and full of beans.

Lucia's typical diet included wholegrain toast with avocado or cheese for breakfast. She would eat a bran muffin or fruit for morning tea. Lunch was a sandwich with chicken or beef and salad. Afternoon tea with her girls included wholegrain crackers with cheese. Dinner was pasta or rice. She didn't have a sweet tooth, so there were no concerns about too much sugar.

Lucia's symptoms of exhaustion, anxiety, puffy face and eyelids, slow bowels and achy joints indicated a problem with her thyroid gland. When I asked if anyone in her family had thyroid issues, she said her mother had Hashimoto's disease and her sister had been diagnosed with hypothyroidism but she didn't know if it had an autoimmune component.

Lucia's blood tests had revealed that her TSH was in the normal range and so her GP hadn't asked for further testing of her thyroid. At one stage, she was even offered medication for anxiety. I ordered tests of Lucia's T3 and T4, and these revealed Hashimoto's, urinary iodine and thyroid antibodies. No wonder she felt depleted.

Lucia's case is not unusual. Each week, I see patients with similar complaints and concerns including puffiness, memory loss and lack of vitality.

My advice to Lucia

In the past, Lucia had chosen good-quality breads made with sourdough, seeds and rye. But each contains gluten. Lucia followed the rebalance and cut out gluten completely.

After painting a hard-core picture of the unsexy, ageing effects of stress blowing out her thyroid and making her fat and unhappy, I convinced Lucia to slow down. The cortisol released due to stress can stimulate the thyroid to work harder. This hormone chaos leads to weight gain, depleted energy and unstable mood. I encouraged Lucia to find moments in her day to rest, sit, enjoy a meal, take a walk and just give in.

Lucia's results

Because of her ongoing chronic tiredness and resulting feelings of failure as a mum, Lucia was motivated to make changes and followed the rebalance strictly. She removed gluten and dairy from her diet and cut out caffeine and alcohol for 28 days. She increased natural iodine by adding dulse flakes to one meal each day, and antioxidants by eating vegetables at every meal. Lucia even joined a meditation class, which at first felt very unnatural to her. For the first six weeks, she hated attending the class, but then the practice began to click. Meditation slowed the constant chatter in her mind – a subtle but relentless driver of stress and increased cortisol. As a result, her cortisol levels went down. Four months on, Lucia told me her energy, inner calm and mental clarity were returning.

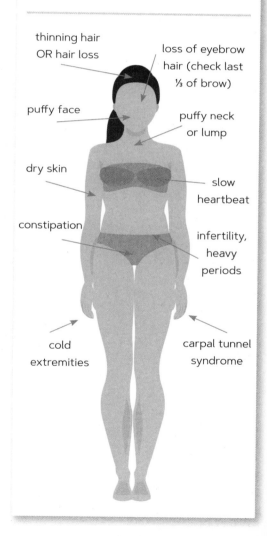

Symptoms of HYPOTHYROIDISM

* Puffiness
* Weight gain
* Poor memory
* Intolerance to cold
* Extreme tiredness

thinning hair OR hair loss

loss of eyebrow hair (check last ⅓ of brow)

puffy face

puffy neck or lump

dry skin

slow heartbeat

constipation

infertility, heavy periods

cold extremities

carpal tunnel syndrome

SEROTONIN

the happy hormone and neurotransmitter

As both a hormone and neurotransmitter, serotonin carries signals along nerves and is responsible for balanced moods, appetite and sleep. Serotonin is a current hot topic for research, particularly into the causes and treatment of depression — one in seven Australians will experience depression in their lifetime. The reasons for depression are complex, but we know serotonin plays a key role in mood.

Serotonin is manufactured both in the brain and the intestines, and 90 per cent of the body's serotonin is located in the gastrointestinal tract. The gut is now referred to as the 'second brain'. With so much serotonin created in the gastrointestinal tract, it makes sense that tummy issues will affect your mood. Even though research is in its infancy, it looks like the brain–gut axis is a two-way street: the gut can affect the brain and the brain affects the gut. Gut bacteria – collectively known as the microbiome – play a significant role in brain chemistry, anxiety and serotonin. The best way to keep gut bacteria in a healthy balance is to cut back on the consumption of excess sugar. Sugar also feeds the yeast fungus known as Candida (see page 200), which can wreak havoc on your gut and causes thrush.

DO YOU HAVE AN ISSUE WITH SEROTONIN?

* Do you tend to be negative?
* Do you worry?
* Do you lack confidence?
* Are you critical of yourself?
* Are you a bit obsessive?
* Are you irritable, impatient, edgy or angry?
* Are you shy or fearful?
* Have you had anxiety attacks or panic attacks?
* Do you get PMS or menopausal moodiness such as tears, anger and/or depression?
* Are you a night owl?
* Do you find it difficult to fall sleep, even when you're tired?
* Do you wake up in the night, have restless or light sleep, or wake up too early in the morning?
* Do you crave sweet or starchy snacks or wine in the late afternoon or evenings but not earlier in the day?
* Do you find relief from any of the above symptoms through exercise?
* Have you had fibromyalgia (unexplained muscle pain) or temporomandibular joint (TMJ) issues (pain, tension, and grinding associated with your jaw)?

If you answered yes to five or more of these questions, you could have a serotonin imbalance. Consult your GP, qualified nutritionist or other health professional for the go-ahead to follow the 28-day Hormone Rebalance. If your symptoms persist, you may need further medical assistance.

HOW TO REBALANCE SEROTONIN

1. Eat well

More than 90 per cent of serotonin is made in the gut, and it makes sense that if your gut is happy and functional, there'll be an improvement in your mood. One of the easiest ways to clean up the gut is to cut out sugary, high-carb processed foods and soft drinks, including diet soft drinks. Preliminary findings suggest a link between drinking diet soft drinks and depression. Foods with a high glycemic index (GI), such as white bread and dried fruits, are also to be avoided. The GI indicates how carbohydrates affect blood glucose levels, and a high GI means the release of glucose is quick. Dried fruit is also high in sugar, even though it's natural sugar. Dried fruit often also contains sulfites used as a preservative. A good intake of healthy fats is also in order.

Another excellent way to improve gut health is to ensure a healthy population of good bacteria by taking a probiotic and eating fermented foods, such as sauerkraut and kimchi. The fermented milk drink kefir also contains healthy bacteria. Once only the province of health food stores, kefir is now widely available. There are dairy-free options including coconut kefir and coconut yoghurt. Try adding 1 tablespoon of kefir to your smoothies.

2. Replace gluten with sweet potatoes and plant protein

The protein in wheat (gluten), rye and barley contains gliadin. This triggers zonulin, which can open the spaces between cells in the stomach, causing intestinal permeability or 'leaky gut'. Many of my clients have reported increased energy, reduced brain fog and less bloating after they remove gluten from their diet. But be aware that products that are marketed as gluten-free can be high in sugar and highly processed. Choose those with the fewest ingredients on the label. As health advocate Michael Pollan says, 'Don't eat anything your great-grandmother wouldn't recognize as food.'

Rather than eating bread and pasta, aim to increase your intake of complex carbohydrates, from foods such as sweet potato and legumes – chickpeas, beans and lentils. In addition to protein, legumes contain complex carbohydrates that are important as brain and muscle fuel. Their fibre content keeps digestion flowing, cleaning your pipes and flattening your tummy.

3. Cut back on alcohol

While serotonin levels rise when we have a drink, over time alcohol depletes levels of the feel-good hormone by interfering with the amino acid tryptophan, which the body needs to produce serotonin. Alcohol also decreases levels of vitamin B, the energy vitamin. We think we feel good, initially anyway, from drinking alcohol because of a short-lived dopamine hit that masks the activities of other neurotransmitters. And we're more likely to eat bad food and skip exercise when we drink.

4. Increase intake of vitamin B12 and iron

The indicators of iron deficiency include hair loss, low energy and depression. The indicators of low vitamin B12 include depression, memory loss and fatigue. A ferritin blood test measures the amount of iron in the body. If your levels are lower than 50 micrograms per litre, you will need to increase your consumption of iron-rich foods or take an iron bisglycinate supplement (see page 224).

Food sources of vitamin B12 include eggs, mushrooms and nutritional yeast. Nutritional yeast is derived from yeast but doesn't contain any live yeast. It looks like grated cheese and has a savoury taste. It can be added to salads and soups – a must-try during the rebalance. Food sources of iron for non-meat eaters include lentils, peas, baked beans, nut butters, hummus, tahini and green leafy vegetables.

5. De-stress

The link between the gut, brain and stress has been demonstrated in one small study by psychologists at Swinburne University of Technology. They sampled the poo of 23 healthy undergraduate students months before they took exams and then during exams, a time when most people feel stressed and the students rated their own stress as high. The researchers measured the students' levels of gut lactic acid bacteria. They found that when the students experienced the perceived stress of taking an exam, there were fewer lactobacilli in their poo sample. We need lactobacilli for the production of serotonin and for good digestion. Low serotonin levels flatten our mood (see page 224 for suggested supplements). One of the best ways to de-stress, exercise and improve vitamin D levels is to walk in fresh air in the sun.

Mood disorders are increasing at an alarming rate. And while anxiety and depression have many causes, research reveals eating nutrient-rich food can improve mental wellbeing.

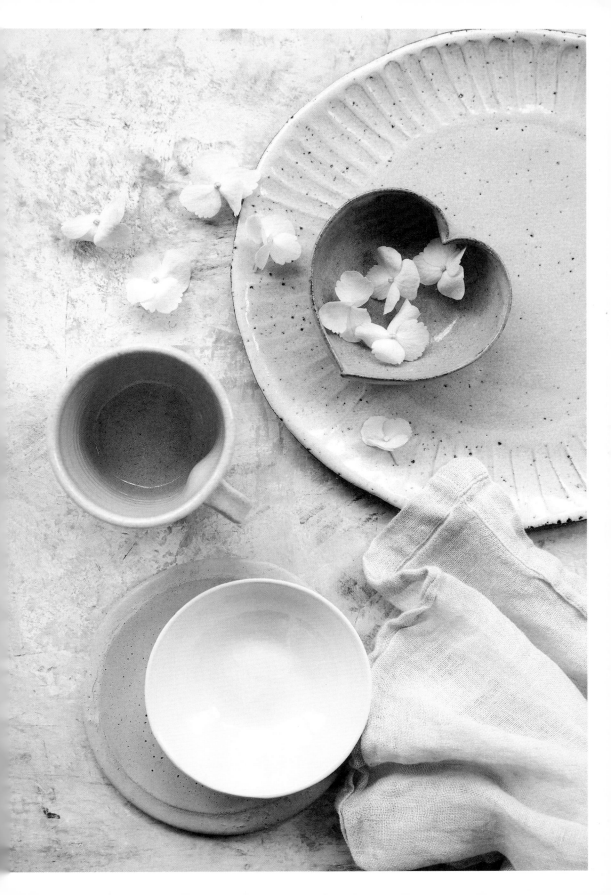

ASHLEY'S ANXIETY

When she was 49, Ashley started to feel anxious and depressed. Her hair was thinning and she had small bald patches on parts of her scalp. As you would expect, Ashley was self-conscious about her appearance and it affected her work and family. She was a lawyer working part time for an insurance company, but she couldn't simply run away and hide. She and her husband had three teenagers, hefty school fees and a mortgage to pay.

Given her age, Ashley thought her symptoms were a sign of perimenopause or menopause, and that perhaps she should just not say anything and simply accept that how she was feeling was just a 'natural part of ageing'.

It really concerns me that many women believe they need to accept subpar energy, vitality and joy because they think they're dealing with menopause. Menopause is a stage, not an illness, and in any case, Ashley's health issues were not menopause-related.

Even though she usually slept for nine or ten hours a night, Ashley didn't wake in the morning feeling refreshed, and this lack of energy continued throughout the day. She was a vegetarian – a practice she undertook five years earlier because of health problems. In one year, she suffered from pneumonia, bronchitis and three bouts of sinusitis which required several rounds of antibiotics. Following this illness, she had tummy issues.

Ashley's typical diet included a cup of tea and Vegemite on toast or a bowl of fruit for breakfast. Morning tea was often a muffin and 'sneaky' diet cola. Lunch was a green salad or salad sandwich and fruit such as grapes, raisins or a banana. Dinner was usually pasta or rice with tomatoes, spinach and other vegetables. Before going to bed, she was in the habit of eating dried fruit to 'keep her bowels moving'.

I'm not opposed to vegan or vegetarian diets as long as they include adequate sources of vitamin B12 and iron. If not, they can lead to anxiety and depression. People who are vegetarian are also at risk of poor lean muscle mass and hair loss. Ashley's blood tests revealed deficiencies in both iron and vitamin B12, levels of which are often not routinely tested by GPs. In my assessment, Ashley's serotonin levels were depleted.

My advice to Ashley

The diet soft drinks that Ashley drank most days were highly likely to be bad for her gut bacteria and to be playing a role in her anxiety by affecting her serotonin levels. The bread and fruits she ate didn't provide lasting fuel for her brain or muscles because they have a high GI. Not only that, the dried fruit was high in sugar even though it was natural sugar. The dried fruit was probably not as good for her as she thought, and her diet was lacking in protein and good fats.

I naturally suggested that she make improvements in all these areas.

Because of her previous antibiotic use, Ashley needed to repopulate her gut with good bacteria through a probiotic and by consuming fermented foods. Because she loved eating veggies, I suggested placing a small tablespoon of kimchi or fermented sauerkraut to the side of eggs or salad. I also encouraged her to drink kefir for healthy bacteria.

Ashley grimaced when I told her to remove gluten from her diet – a common reaction when I ask someone to remove an item they love. It's only when I tell them how it will impact their weight, energy and mood that I can get them to commit. I suggested to Ashley that there would be no harm in finding out how she felt when she cut out gluten.

Instead of bread, Ashley's menu featured sweet potato (roasted, toasted, baked, mashed or as bread) and legumes, which provided much-needed slow-release carbohydrates for fuelling her brain and body, and also provided lots of fibre to keep her gut bacteria happy and her digestion running smoothly. And while she loved to drink wine, she loved feeling good even more, and so committed to only drinking two glasses of wine on weekends and never during the week.

Ashley's stress levels were very high because of work and family responsibilities. She committed to walking outside for 30 minutes three times a week, to unwind while exercising and boosting her vitamin D levels. I also suggested she introduce stress-reducing exercises such as yoga or Pilates, and that she take calming herbs and supplements.

Ashley's results

Ashley and I worked together for more than fifteen months. She increased her intake of foods high in vitamin B12 and in each meal included a plant protein or slow-release carb, with veggies, sauce, pesto or dip to make it more appealing. Every day, she ate iron-rich food (see the list on page 224). Sweet potato was her go-to substitute when she craved bread, and her favourite breakfast was warm sweet potato with goat's cheese. Months later, when I bumped into Ashley at the local yoga studio, she smiled as she tossed around a full head of hair. 'Look at this. Look at me,' she said proudly. Her eyes were bright, her hair thick and shiny, and you could feel her renewed energy. It took my breath away.

Anxiety is debilitating. It robs us of sleep, careers and joy. As a first step, ensure adequate intake of B12 vitamins and iron.

TESTOSTERONE
the hormone of vitality

Testosterone is one of the sex hormones and is described as the hormone of vitality and self-confidence. And even though it's mostly associated with men, women also need testosterone, although not as much as men. One of the main reasons for female infertility may be excess testosterone. It also affects sex drive: too little causes low libido in women and men. The good news is that changes to your diet and lifestyle can bring this hormone back into balance.

MEN: DO YOU HAVE AN ISSUE WITH TESTOSTERONE?

* Are you losing body hair or shrinking in height?
* Is it difficult for you to build lean muscle mass, despite exercising regularly?
* Do you lack energy and feel tired?
* Do you have decreased endurance or strength?
* Are you sad or grumpy?
* Do you feel depressed or anxious?
* Do you have decreased sex drive?
* Is your erection less strong?
* Do you have man boobs?
* Do you struggle to lose weight?
* Have you been diagnosed with low bone density or osteoporosis?

WOMEN: DO YOU HAVE AN ISSUE WITH TESTOSTERONE?

* Do you feel exhausted even after eight hours of sleep?
* Are you gaining weight?
* Do you have reduced libido and vaginal dryness?
* Do you feel unstable and lack mental clarity?
* Have you been diagnosed with low bone density or osteoporosis?
* Do you have irregular periods but are not perimenopausal or menopausal?
* Is your hair thinning or falling out?

If you answered yes to three or more of these questions, you could have a testosterone imbalance. Consult your GP, qualified nutritionist or other health professional for the go-ahead to follow the 28-day Hormone Rebalance. If your symptoms persist, you may need further medical assistance.

HOW TO REBALANCE TESTOSTERONE

1. Eat well
Testosterone levels can be boosted by eating nutritious foods. Vegetables should play a leading role in every meal because they're full of fibre, vitamins and antioxidants,

and they make you feel full. Watch your snacking and stick to the healthy suggestions on pages 96–7.

2. Cut down on alcohol

Alcohol lowers testosterone levels. Many people use alcohol to help them unwind and to take the edge off a stressful day. And while it feels as though a drink or two helps you relax, knocking back a couple of schooners with dinner diminishes the quality of sleep. Drinking in the evening and before bed stops the body resting compared with drinking at other times of day. One of the biggest problems is a reduction in REM sleep, the deepest and most restorative phase. Men who drink excessive alcohol have impaired testosterone production and shrinkage of the testes. I know it can be a bitter pill to swallow, particularly with the Australian drinking culture, but because alcohol drops testosterone, it affects mood and energy. Alcohol also affects the release of other hormones related to men's sexual function and fertility. Enlarged breasts are common in heavy drinkers because alcohol converts testosterone into oestrogen.

3. Get good-quality sleep

Too little sleep alters metabolism and hormone function. In one study, a group of healthy older men wore a wristband as they slept to measure their testosterone levels. Those who slept for only four hours had about half the testosterone of those who slept for eight hours. The longer men sleep, the greater their testosterone levels – it's

that simple. In another study, lack of sleep lowered testosterone, causing lower libido, lower strength, poor concentration and fatigue – the equivalent of ten to fifteen years of ageing.

Some ways to increase sleep include:

* reducing sugar consumption
* limiting your caffeine intake to one coffee per day
* taking magnesium (see below) or the sleep hormone melatonin
* not drinking liquids after 6 pm, to minimise the need for a toilet break in the middle of the night.

4. Increase nutrient uptake

I prefer that food be the main source of nutrients, but in some cases there's a need for supplements. Vitamin C and garlic increase levels of nitric oxide – a key signalling molecule for blood flow, artery dilation and erectile function. Magnesium is the eleventh most abundant mineral in the body and controls more than 300 bodily functions. Deficiencies in this vital mineral can lead to lower levels of testosterone. Zinc (40 mg a day) is also important for testosterone production, and research suggests that taking supplements for as little as six weeks can improve testosterone levels. Vitamin D is a steroid hormone that assists with sperm production and increases testosterone, which is important for a healthy sex life. In one study, overweight men who took vitamin D supplements for a year had a significant increase in testosterone.

DAVID SIDESTEPS DIABETES

David, 54, runs the IT section at a large firm. He'd recently visited his GP who took some tests and the results weren't good. His blood glucose reading of 10.5 mml/L indicated prediabetes, which was his wake-up call to change his eating habits. He didn't want to become a statistic.

David said he felt tired, was gaining weight and was always busy at work. His partner had prompted him to see me, suggesting he needed a midlife change rather than a midlife crisis. As with many men, David knew his mood, energy and sleep could be improved but he didn't know where to start. He didn't want to be overweight and he certainly didn't want to be pre-diabetic. His hectic work life matched the many professionals I see each week. Even though they are time-poor, they desire good health.

David's diet was high in carbohydrates, with minimal protein consumed throughout the day. His sugar intake was high and his vegetable intake was very low. The demands of his busy job meant frequent 'grab and go' food choices. On the plus side, his alcohol consumption was lower than the average 'Aussie bloke', consisting of 2–3 drinks per week. This was a bonus because alcohol can create a hormone rollercoaster. For exercise, David enjoyed walking but not to the level that it could shift excess weight from his 110 kg frame. We discussed the benefits of high intensity interval training or HIIT (see page 78). Evidence suggests HIIT improves the effectiveness of insulin receptors.

As men age, it's normal for their testosterone levels to decline. But there are problems if the rate accelerates, particularly if insulin resistance is also part of the story. Many men aged over 50 have trouble with their blood-sugar and glucose levels and are often pre-diabetic. It's the case for many women as well. When insulin resistance becomes part of the health history, hormonal chaos is generally also implicated. Insulin affects the function of both testosterone and oestrogen in the body. High insulin can also switch off the functioning of leptin – a scenario to avoid. This is because leptin signals when we've had enough to eat. Some people can consume 5–6 meals a day and still feel hungry because their leptin signals are not working properly.

As I explain to many men, carrying extra weight is a problem because an enzyme called aromatase in fat cells converts testosterone into oestrogen. Low levels of testosterone and too much oestrogen can cause 'man boobs'. This wasn't something David had to deal with but I often discuss this with patients and they really listen and take action when they hear the words 'man boobs'. If you're overweight, you're also more likely to experience poor moods, lower energy and concentration and reduced muscle tone. Nearly 40 per cent of obese men aged over 45 have low blood levels of testosterone.

Another issue associated with extra weight is high cholesterol. David was smart to want to reduce his levels through changing his diet because cholesterol medication can have unwanted side effects including painful muscle cramps and reduced sex drive.

Men over the age of 50 are advised to have their prostate specific-antigen (PSA) levels checked. These days, a growing number of younger men are being diagnosed with prostate cancer and it's the type of cancer they will die from, rather than die with.

My advice to David

David represents the 'new normal', which is actually an unhealthy normal. He had to improve his nutrition, lose weight and increase his exercise to balance insulin, testosterone and cortisol. The first order of business was to boost his vegetable intake. I told him this doesn't mean eating broccoli every night. He could spice things up. Yes, steamed broccoli is on the menu, but with added flavours such as Moroccan spices or chilli oil.

I told him he didn't have to worry about portion sizes and I promised he wouldn't feel hungry. After one week following the rebalance, David told me he'd had headaches for the first few days but liked that there was no portion control. His headaches were a symptom of sudden sugar withdrawal.

David's results

Two months after starting the rebalance, David had lost 9 kilograms. He visited his GP and sent me this email: 'I've been very strict at observing what I learned in your program. As a result, my cholesterol has returned to a "normal" zone, my blood glucose went from 10.5 to 6.5. My prostate-specific antigen (PSA) levels are lower than they were two years ago, which my doctor said was extraordinary for a 54-year-old bloke. Every other test was back to normal readings. My blood pressure reading was the lowest it's been in ten years. He took the reading twice to ensure it was accurate. Frankly, he was astounded. It'd be fair to say that when I first joined the program, I was a ticking time bomb. You did promise you'd turn me into a "lean, mean, sexy machine", but more importantly I think you may have saved my life – all because I'm good at following the five simple rules [for food combining] you gave me [see page 88]. I'm treating this as a long-term project and feel for the first time in probably twenty years that it's actually achievable with the tools you've given me. I'm also blessed to have a supportive partner in my life who fully embraces the process. I have much to be grateful for. Thank you, Michele, from the bottom of my much healthier heart.' My own heart filled with joy, as it does with every client who transforms their health and makes it the norm.

LEPTIN
the hunger hormone

Leptin is the current contender for most popular hormone of the year award. Across the world, endocrinologists, neuroscientists and psychologists are studying the processes by which leptin affects fat storage. Leptin helps inhibit hunger and regulates energy balance. It's secreted by fat cells and sends a signal to the brain so we stop eating when the body has enough fuel in storage.

When working well, leptin triggers the hypothalamus to lower appetite, allowing the body to dip into its fat stores. People who are obese produce too much leptin and the receptors stop working, causing leptin resistance. Leptin fails to send the 'I'm full' signal to the brain, which thinks there's not enough fat stored. You might have all the willpower in the world, but if your levels of leptin are unbalanced, they win every time. One of the complications in losing weight is that lower leptin levels can trigger an increase in appetite and food cravings, making weight loss more challenging.

Leptin can be suppressed by eating too much sugar. In particular, it's affected by too much fructose, which is used as a sweetener and can also be listed as agave (75 per cent fructose), crystalline fructose and high-fructose corn syrup. In addition, when table sugar (sucrose) is broken down

in our digestive system, the products are half glucose and half fructose. Most Australians consume up to 75 grams of fructose a day but we shouldn't have more than 25 grams per day. If you eat two pieces of fruit with 10 grams of fructose each, this won't cause liver damage, but it's a different story with soft drinks, cordials, cereals and sweetened yoghurts. Fructose is metabolised by the liver. If there's too much fructose, the liver has to work overtime, and excess fructose is stored as fat. High insulin levels, triggering storage of sugar as fat, trump leptin signals saying we're full – the brain doesn't see there's plenty of stored energy and sends out hunger pangs.

DO YOU HAVE A LEPTIN IMBALANCE?

* Are you 7 kilograms or more overweight, with most of the fat around your belly?
* Do you feel hungry all the time and not satisfied after eating?
* Do you get less than seven or eight hours' sleep?
* Do you feel stressed? High cortisol levels lead to leptin resistance.
* Has your exercise routine fallen off the rails?
* Do you have strong cravings for sweet foods?

* Do you become a human vacuum cleaner after 5 pm?
* Do you have menopausal puffiness, especially around your waist?
* Do you have 'nana arms' – or flapping under the triceps muscle?
* Do you have joint aches and pains that you never had before – knee or shoulder bursitis, or arthritis?

If you answered yes to five or more of these questions, you could have leptin imbalance. Consult your GP, qualified nutritionist or other health professional for the go-ahead to follow the 28-day Hormone Rebalance. If your symptoms persist, you may need further medical assistance.

HOW TO REBALANCE LEPTIN

1. Eat slowly, eat well

Try to finish eating dinner at least three hours before bed and to stop eating each meal when slightly less than full. When you eat slowly, you know when you've had just enough and not too much, just like Goldilocks. Also try to ensure you eat about 20 grams of protein at breakfast. One egg has 7–9 grams of protein. If you add avocado and flaxseeds, you're almost at 20 grams. Another suggestion is smoked salmon and avocado on a bed of spinach. Quality fats, such as those in avocado and salmon, are also important to stabilise leptin. Consider a pea protein shake, but only if you're finding it too difficult to obtain adequate protein from your food – you know I like to take a food-first approach with nutrition. Limit but don't cut out all

carbs. During the rebalance, you'll obtain your carbs from starchy vegetables, non-gluten grains and low-sugar fruit. I call them slow carbs or smart carbs. Slow because they're absorbed slowly by the body and don't cause a spike in blood sugar. Smart because they're packed with fibre, which makes you feel full.

2. Get a good night's sleep

When you place your body under stress, your cortisol levels go up and stay up, which increases your risk of developing insulin resistance and leptin resistance. Even if you believe you can function on fewer than eight hours a night, science tells a different story. Studies reveal a link between sleep, weight, insulin resistance and decreased leptin. And because you're awake for longer, the body sends a signal that it needs more fuel in the tank – hello, hunger pangs.

A summary of 36 sleep studies showed that sleeping fewer hours reduces leptin levels and elevates its opposing hormone, ghrelin, which increases appetite levels. Not only that, the studies suggest that when we're tired, we're less likely to exercise. The link between sleep deprivation and weight gain appears to be especially strong in children. In one study, young men who slept for only four hours over two consecutive nights had an 18 per cent reduction in leptin and 28 per cent increase in ghrelin. Sleep deprivation leads to food cravings, particularly for sweet and starchy foods, perhaps because the brain is fuelled by glucose. When we don't get enough sleep, our brain doesn't respond to insulin telling us we have fuel on board, and it craves sugar for sustenance. If you give in to these cravings, you'll gain weight.

3. Limit fructose

If your leptin levels are high, cut back on fructose. Regardless of leptin levels, always avoid high-fructose corn syrup (which is relatively rare in Australian processed foods anyway) and eat as little sugar as possible. The rebalance allows two serves of low-sugar fruit such as berries a day, but if you're leptin-resistant, you should avoid high-sugar fruits such as mangoes, bananas, other tropical fruit and watermelon. Rats fed a 60 per cent fructose diet for six months developed fructose-induced leptin resistance. Another reason to avoid fructose is that it messes with the liver, which has to be in top shape for hormone balance.

4. Increase fibre

Most Australians don't eat enough fibre, which is vital for weight loss. Many only eat half the recommended 25–35 grams per day. Fibre helps us feel full and satisfied, maintains bowel health and a healthy weight, lowers cholesterol and regulates blood sugar. Vegetables and legumes are good sources, and you can add 2 teaspoons of ground flaxseeds to smoothies, salads or soups. To avoid tummy upsets, add fibre to your diet slowly. If your bowels can tolerate it and aren't loose, add fibre twice a day. If your stools are loose, reduce your fibre intake first, then increase it again slowly. When you're adding fibre, you must be drinking more water. Otherwise you can end up with a big ball of fibre in your bowel.

You might have all the willpower in the world, but if your leptin levels are unbalanced, they win every time.

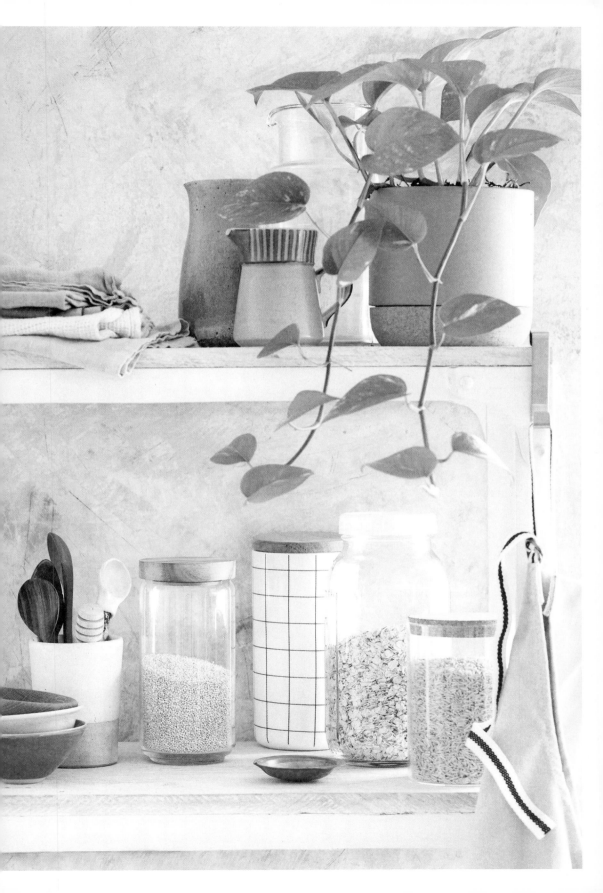

TRACY IS THIN, TIRED AND HUNGRY

Tracy has a very complex relationship with food. As a teenager, she became obsessed with calorie counting and progressed to full-blown eating disorders when she was seventeen.

Now 36, Tracy is married with two children under the age of five and works as a physical education teacher. Over the past six years, Tracy had gained 1–2 kilograms a year, despite restricting her calories. Even with this weight gain, she was teetering at the low end of a healthy weight. The food group that was the mainstay of her diet was fruit. Always feeling hungry and often light-headed, she knew this was an unsustainable way of eating.

Tracy chose fruit for several reasons. After years of taking antibiotics for sinus and respiratory infections, she worried about her vitamin levels. She also liked the fibre in fruit because when she was bulimic, her bowels came to a standstill. And she was convinced that a low-fat diet and weight-loss teas kept her thin in her early twenties. Fruit matched the fat-free approach.

Tracy's diet included two skim-milk fruit smoothies for breakfast and lunch. Morning and afternoon tea were fruit. Dinner was boiled pumpkin or sweet potato with lentils, chickpeas or brown rice. She told me, 'I feel like a failure who's always starving.' I told her many people feel like this, including me, and that the scales only offer us a physical measurement. They don't reveal your worth as a person. I insisted she stop weighing herself twice a day, and to stop beating herself up.

In my assessment, Tracy had leptin sensitivity that made her feel hungry. While most people with leptin sensitivity are overweight, it can also occur in people who are underweight. Because Tracy had two children under the age of five, her sleep was often disturbed, and lack of sleep increases the levels of cortisol, which contributes to leptin sensitivity. And even though fruit is healthy, she was eating far too much of it. Instead what she really needed was slow carbs and sustaining protein.

My advice to Tracy

In addition to the rebalance, Tracy had to finish eating dinner at least three hours before bedtime and to finish each meal when slightly less than full. She also had to ensure she ate around 20 grams of protein at breakfast, and to limit her consumption of carbs without cutting them out altogether. I asked Tracy to make sleep a key focus, to cut down on the fruit and to increase her intake of other fibre sources. Because Tracy is a PE teacher, she was already exercising regularly, and this would assist her in achieving healthy leptin levels.

Tracy's results

Tracy's nutritionally balanced diet boosted her mood and energy. With each meal, she balanced protein, complex carbs and quality fats. Rather than snacking on fruit, she had a handful of nuts. This stabilised her blood sugar levels and eventually her leptin levels. Sleep was more of a challenge, but she worked on creating a restful environment in her bedroom. Because of her past eating disorder, Tracy's results were slow and steady, but she persisted and succeeded in achieving good energy levels and maintaining her weight without feeling hungry all the time. Tracy is now healthy and vibrant, and is embarking on studying positive psychology.

This plan is based on nourishment, not punishment. It's about smart carbs, not no carbs.

OESTROGEN

the protective hormone

In women, oestrogen is involved in menstruation, pregnancy, sex drive, healthy skin, cognitive function, bone health and lubrication of the joints, eyes and vagina. If oestrogen levels are too low, this causes insomnia, low libido, mood swings and dry skin. If too high, it can cause weight gain, menstrual issues, premenstrual syndrome (PMS), cystic breasts, fibroids and some cancers.

Oestrogen can also be a factor in migraine headaches, particularly just before the start of your period when oestrogen levels drop. Ideally, you want a fine balance between oestrogen and progesterone, its partner hormone. In some cases, women have too much oestrogen when they're young and not enough after menopause. This happened to me and to many of my friends. Because oestrogen is anti-inflammatory, when levels drop during menopause, some women feel like they've been hit by a truck. Menopause is a natural part of ageing, and if your adrenal glands are healthy, they can produce some protective oestrogen – another reason to keep your adrenal glands and stress under control and in balance.

Oestrogen also plays an important role in men, affecting testosterone, bone density, skin and collagen health, sexual function, cardiovascular disease and cholesterol.

In men, too much oestrogen can cause enlarged breasts, erectile dysfunction and infertility.

In men and women, excess body fat increases oestrogen production. A diet high in refined carbohydrates such as breads, cakes, cereals and pasta raises blood sugar and insulin levels, and increases body fat.

Because oestrogen affects both men and women, I have included male and female case studies in this section. Pick and choose the information from below that is relevant to your sex.

EXCESS OESTROGEN AND PMS

PMS usually happens in the week before your period, due to an imbalance between oestrogen levels and progesterone levels. The symptoms include irritability, anxiety, fluid retention, heavy periods and weight gain on the hips. Eating a whole-food diet helps the body eliminate excess hormones that potentially add to PMS – namely oestrogen. Excess oestrogen is broken down in the liver, where it can affect other important liver functions. It's why limiting or removing alcohol is so important for those who experience painful PMS symptoms. My clients are amazed that in just a few weeks they could clean up their liver. Symptoms of low progesterone (and thus oestrogen excess) include infertility, low libido, weepiness, PMS, hair loss and sleep issues. Progesterone is a soothing hormone and affected by stress, thyroid dysfunction and insulin resistance. When the body is excessively stressed, cortisol can steal progesterone.

The causes of excess oestrogens include:

* **xenoestrogens** – These oestrogen-mimicking chemicals are found in pesticides, dry-cleaning chemicals, plastics, nail polish, perfumes, birth-control pills and more. I pride myself on being a nutritionist who lives in the real world, and I don't like to see everything as toxic, but the more I research endocrine disruptors, the more alarmed I become. Be aware and do the best you can. I use all-natural lipstick and hair-colouring. After dry-cleaning clothes, I air them outside before returning them to the wardrobe.
* **gut-flora imbalance** – When gut bacteria are unbalanced, toxins aren't cleared and can be reabsorbed. Two gut-flora disruptors are excessive antibiotics and sugar. If you have to take antibiotics, repopulate your gut with good bacteria by taking a probiotic or eating prebiotic and probiotic foods such as kefir, sauerkraut, kimchi, unflavoured yoghurt, gherkins and apple cider vinegar. Sugar feeds bad gut bacteria, helping them take over in the gut and have a party. Avoid hidden sugars and eat only naturally occurring sugars in fruits and vegetables.
* **liver overload** – When the liver is working optimally, it detoxifies the body naturally. Keep your alcohol intake to a minimum, eat fibrous vegetables, avoid taking excessive paracetamol, and choose foods that are high in vitamin B, selenium and amino acids (see page 113).
* **excess weight** – Fat (adipose tissue) can create a form of oestrogen called oestrone, which can impair healthy oestrogen and affect fertility. It could also contribute to polycystic ovary syndrome (PCOS).
* **low progesterone** – As women age, their progesterone levels decrease and this can lead to oestrogen excess. Increase your progesterone levels by eating grass-fed butter and free-range eggs. Magnesium helps break down oestrogen. Vitamin C increases progesterone. If you can't source sufficient vitamins from your food, use supplements, but always use food for nutrition first.
* **perimenopause** – You can be perimenopausal for up to ten years before true menopause (see overleaf) hits. During this time, oestrogen and progesterone levels swing like kids in a playground. The healthier you are, the less likely you are to be afflicted by fluctuations in mood and energy.
* **constipation** – Keep your fibre intake up. You don't want oestrogen to be reabsorbed after the liver has filtered it.

OESTROGEN DECLINE AND MENOPAUSE

Menopause occurs when the monthly release of oestrogen declines significantly. Official menopause is when menstruation has ceased for twelve continuous months. Signs of oestrogen decline are poor memory, loss of elastin in the skin, decreased libido, dry eyes and vagina, and poor sleep quality. Menopause causes a decline in melatonin, the sleep hormone, which regulates body temperature. After menopause, the body doesn't process carbohydrates as efficiently and tends to store the excess as fat. It's a good reason to look after your adrenal glands. If they're healthy, they'll still pump out a little oestrogen even after menopause.

Women shouldn't suffer in menopause. If you're struggling, seek the advice of your GP or functional medicine doctor; they could help you explore bio-identical hormones and in some cases conventional hormone replacement therapy (HRT). Seek out phytoestrogen-rich foods such as fennel, celery, buckwheat, brown rice, sesame seeds, caraway seeds, sunflower seeds, sprouted seeds, mung beans, chickpeas, garlic, red onions, yams, organic tempeh and miso.

WOMEN: DO YOU HAVE AN OESTROGEN IMBALANCE?

* Have you been diagnosed with fibroids or ovarian cysts?
* Do you tend to gain weight easily?
* Are PMS or heavy menstrual bleeding a monthly occurrence?
* Do you retain water and get swollen fingers and feet?
* Are you often irritable and anxious?
* Do you bloat easily?
* Do you have sugar cravings?
* Do you get breast tenderness, cysts or enlarged cup size every month?
* Do you eat conventionally raised meat (not organic or pasture-fed) every week?
* Do you have hot flushes or night sweats?
* Do you have difficulty sleeping?
* Do you have dry eyes, skin, and hair?
* Is sex painful from lack of lubrication?
* Are you forgetful?
* Have you lost your libido?
* Do you often experience low energy?
* Have your periods stopped?

MEN: DO YOU HAVE AN OESTROGEN IMBALANCE?

* Has your libido declined?
* Have you noticed a change in erectile function?
* Do you have enlarged breasts?
* Have you had urinary tract symptoms associated with benign enlarged prostate?
* Has your abdominal fat increased?
* Have you noticed a loss in muscle mass?

* Are you suffering from emotional disturbances or depression?
* Have you been diagnosed with type 2 diabetes?

If you answered yes to three or more of these questions, you could have an oestrogen imbalance. Consult your GP, qualified nutritionist or other health professional for the go-ahead to follow the 28-day Hormone Rebalance. If your symptoms persist, you may need further medical assistance.

WOMEN: HOW TO REBALANCE OESTROGEN

1 . Avoid coffee and diet drinks

In one study, women who drank two or more cups of coffee a day, or four cans of cola a day, were twice as likely to develop endometriosis as other women. Diet cola also contains caffeine, and research suggests that the chemicals used as sweeteners in diet drinks, such as aspartame and sucralose, increase insulin levels and activation of intestinal sweet taste receptors. And here comes the cascade effect – increased insulin affects levels of oestrogen, progesterone and testosterone. Insulin resistance also influences weight, with extra glucose converted to fat. In short, you don't want a bar of it. I insist that you not only remove diet drinks from your life completely, but you run from them. After the rebalance, you can drink coffee in moderation.

2. Take care of your liver

One way to do this is to be discerning when using medications such as paracetamol. Its overuse can be harmful to your liver and cause fatty liver issues (see page 113). As we age, progesterone decreases and oestrogen can become disproportionately higher – especially if our liver doesn't function optimally. If not cleared, oestrogen can be reabsorbed in the body, causing oestrogen excess. It means a sluggish liver, weight gain and brain fog. Another way to care for your liver is to keep to a moderate alcohol intake, and never drink without eating, which places greater strain on the liver (see also point 4).

3. Eat more fibre

Bowel movements excrete toxins and excess oestrogen, so it's important to be regular. Assist the process by increasing the amount of fibre in your diet. Sprinkle whole flaxseeds (also called linseeds) over your breakfast, vegetables or salads or, if that doesn't appeal, add ½–1 teaspoon of whole flaxseeds to a glass of water and, as you drink, chew on the flaxseeds. Drink it 20 minutes before breakfast or lunch every day. Fibre makes you feel full and satisfied, so you won't go searching for more food. Flaxseeds are also packed with omega-3 fatty acids that assist with hormone and skin health, insulin sensitivity and inflammation.

4. Eat liver-cleansing vegetables as often as possible

Boost your liver function by eating cruciferous veggies such as broccoli, brussels sprouts, cauliflower, cabbage,

kale, turnip and bok choy. These vegetables are high in glucosinolates, which the body turns into compounds that help decrease oestrogen levels and assist in liver detoxification. Steam, stir-fry or bake your veggies – I don't mind how you prepare them. To mix up the flavours, add spices.

5. Cut out fried foods

Fried and fatty foods increase oestrogen levels. Most fried foods are cooked in partially hydrogenated oils that raise LDL or bad cholesterol and lower HDL or good cholesterol. Remember, we want hormone balance with the Goldilocks effect: not too high and not too low. An increase in cholesterol can affect the level of oestrogen circulating in the body, and some of the cholesterol produced in the liver can be converted into oestrogen.

6. Cut down on meat

One of the reasons red meat is eliminated during the first half of the rebalance is that eating red meat may increase oestrogen levels and excess oestrogen stops us from getting lean. It's also a risk factor for endometriosis. In week 3, lamb is back on the menu and in week 4, you can eat other red meat again. Where possible, buy grass-fed or organic meat. In Australia, around 40 per cent of cattle are grain-finished in feedlots, during which time they are fed hormone growth promotants (HGPs), naturally occurring or synthetic hormones that fatten up the cattle more quickly.

7. Exercise more

Exercise has been shown to reduce overly high oestrogen levels in young women and maintain oestrogen levels in older women.

MEN: HOW TO REBALANCE OESTROGEN

1. Lose weight with diet and exercise

As we've seen, the enzyme aromatase converts testosterone to oestrogen and is found in fat cells. The more fat in the body, particularly in the gut, the more aromatase to convert powerful and protective testosterone into oestrogen. Low testosterone can cause fatigue, low libido and loss of muscle mass. A loss of lean muscle and increase in fat tissue increases aromatase levels.

2. Pack your plate with veggies

Eat as many veggies as you can, particularly cruciferous vegetables such as broccoli, cauliflower, cabbage, brussels sprouts and bok choy. Also helpful for oestrogen metabolism are fish, eggs, spinach, beetroot and quinoa to assist detoxification.

3. Limit your alcohol intake

Alcohol makes the body produce more oestrogen (see page 113).

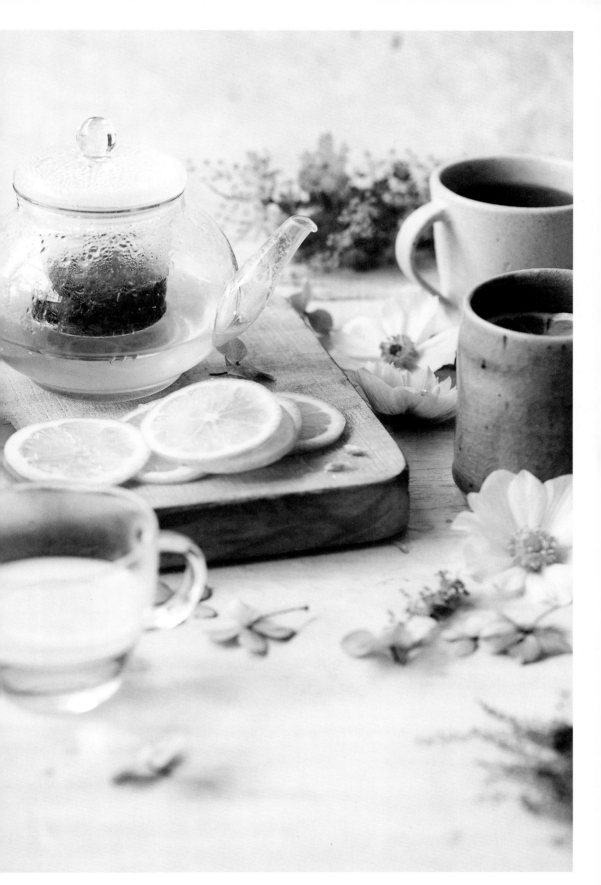

JUSTINE'S WEIGHT GAIN AND ENDOMETRIOSIS

Justine, 41, is a successful dress designer with a passion for vintage fabrics. She is married without children. As with most people who work in an office, Justine sits at a desk for most of her day, and over the years she's fallen victim to 'kilo creep' — a slowly and steady weight gain. But it wasn't until she got a diagnosis of mild endometriosis that she decided it was time to modify her diet and lifestyle. Her commitment to make changes was bolstered by an aunt and a colleague being diagnosed with breast cancer.

Endometriosis occurs when the uterine lining grows in other parts of the body, such as the fallopian tubes or ovaries. Each month this tissue responds to the same hormones that regulate the menstrual cycle and release blood; 75 per cent of women with endometriosis have painful periods or pelvic pain. The cause is unknown but there is speculation that a rise in this condition is related to excess oestrogen in the body. In addition to mild endometriosis, Justine had fibrocystic or lumpy breasts, which is another sign of excess oestrogen. Being overweight also contributes to excess oestrogen, because fat cells make and secrete the hormone. Justine's method to combat the pain from endometriosis was to pop paracetamol, especially before and during her period.

A typical breakfast for Justine included a flat-white coffee and eggs on toast. Lunch was a chicken salad or chicken sandwich. Afternoon tea was a flat-white coffee or diet soft drink or artificially sweetened flavoured sparkling water. Red meat was often on the menu at dinner, along with a couple of glasses of wine. On some nights, Justine 'saved' calories by having a 'liquid dinner' of just wine. This approach to weight management is harmful but more common than you might expect. On the plus side, Justine didn't have a sweet tooth.

Four years earlier, Justine's doctor had said she had irritable bowel syndrome (IBS) and there wasn't anything she could do about it. IBS has, however, been linked with vitamin D deficiency, and Justine's blood tests were in the normal range except for her vitamin D. I suggested she use a vitamin D/vitamin K2 oral spray once a day to boost her levels.

My advice to Justine

It was clear to me that Justine had an issue with her oestrogen levels. This was indicated not only by her medical conditions but her diet. Caffeine (in coffee and diet colas), dairy, red meat and alcohol often worsen symptoms of endometriosis, especially inflammation. Justine needed to turn to healthier options to stay hydrated and use good food rather than a caffeine kick for an energy boost.

I also suggested cutting back on paracetamol. Justine's liver had to be in top shape to remove excess oestrogen – a risk factor for breast cancer, cystic breasts, endometriosis, fibroids, cancers and thyroid suppression. One obvious area for improvement was Justine's alcohol intake, but she was reluctant to give up all alcohol, so we did a deal. During the rebalance, she could drink one glass of red wine with food, but that was it. One glass all week. After the 28 days, she was allowed one or two glasses of wine on no more than three to four nights a week, and always with food. If it was a night when she was fasting (see page 156), alcohol was banned.

Justine needed to increase fibre intake, and I suggested she use whole flaxseeds as one way to do this. Eating whole flaxseeds helps you slow down and chew your food. If flaxseeds are not properly chewed, they come out whole, which means you haven't absorbed their nutrients. It was important for Justine to increase her vegetable intake too, not only for fibre but also because vegetables reduce oestrogen levels. I especially stressed the need for her to increase her intake of cruciferous vegetables.

I also advised her to exercise more, because women who exercise regularly have a lower risk of endometriosis.

Justine's results

Justine's disciplined approach was rewarded: she lost 3 kilograms during the rebalance and an additional 2.5 kilograms over the following three months. She said

the plan was easy to follow and she didn't feel hungry. She even asked me if she should stop drinking wine altogether! I said if the distress of not having a glass or two of red wine would make her super-cranky and intolerable, then the answer was no. In a perfect health world, no one would ingest any caffeine, alcohol, unhealthy fats or preservatives. But we don't live in a perfect world, and there are many stages to good health. Justine continued to apply the five food-combining rules (see page 88). She loved eating red meat and dairy, and so decided to spend extra money on grass-fed or organically grown meats and organic dairy. She also had only a small amount of dairy.

At the end of the rebalance, Justine decided to stay off gluten. She believed the reason for her significantly reduced pain levels was her new eating plan, and I agree with her. Many people are unaware of just how flat they feel until they follow this plan. They suddenly have more energy, clearer brain function, and a greater desire for exercise and even for sex. Justine connected her health dots and noticed her tummy stopped puffing up in the morning after she cut out wheat. She didn't look slightly pregnant any more, whereas before, 90 minutes after eating pasta, wholegrain bread or a bowl of cereal, her tummy was puffed up and painful.

Justine was now exercising every day, even if it was just a brisk walk with girlfriends before work. She reported that her energy levels had never been this good.

JOHN REGAINS HIS YOUTH

John, 56, is married with three teenage children. Eleven years ago he had a career change — leaving his job as a hands-on electrician to manage his own electrician business. This means that rather than visit sites throughout the day, carrying ladders and crawling under floors, he now sits behind a desk. His working days are longer and more stressful, and he has less time for exercise and healthy eating.

You can probably guess what happened to John's weight over that time. Slowly but surely he added several kilos, particularly across his stomach. There were signs of man boobs as well. He lost muscle mass, felt tired and his libido was in decline. John's blood tests showed slightly elevated prostate-specific antigen (PSA) and mild insulin resistance. He said his father had been diagnosed with prostate cancer.

John's typical breakfast was a cup of tea with sourdough toast, margarine and jam. By mid-morning, he was hungry so he ate more toast with coffee. Lunch from the local takeaway was often a sandwich or fish and chips and a juice. During the afternoon, he snacked on biscuits or the lollies kept in an open bowl in the office kitchen. Dinner was meat and three veg with a slice of bread and margarine on the side. He had a weakness for ice cream, cake, sausage rolls and pies – food his three teenage boys could still eat

without putting on weight. He often drank wine and beers.

John's symptoms of enlarged breasts, abdominal fat, tiredness, loss of muscle, increased PSA levels and insulin resistance suggested excess oestrogen. The main causes of increased oestrogen are age and increased body fat. And the reason men need to pay attention to oestrogen is that it regulates testosterone, brain function, bone health, cardiovascular health and sexual function. Research also points to a link between excess oestrogen in men and prostate cancer. When oestrogen levels are out of whack, it increases the risk of degenerative diseases such as stroke and coronary artery disease.

My advice to John

I told John he could reduce his levels of oestrogen by losing weight through the rebalance and regular exercise. John committed to three high-intensity interval training cycle classes a week along with weight training.

My main dietary advice to John was to pack his plate with veggies, particularly cruciferous vegetables. And instead of lollies, I suggested he stock the office kitchen with brazil nuts, almonds and walnuts, which would help raise his testosterone levels. I also suggested he replace margarine with butter. Margarine contains partially hydrogenated fatty acids that can damage arteries and are linked with insulin resistance. Gluten also affects oestrogen levels and I encouraged John to give up bread and other wheat products.

John's results

John was determined not to become an 'old man' and have a 'dad bod', especially for his children. Over ten months, he shed 10 kilograms, mostly from his belly and his man boobs. At my practice, the people with the best long-term success at maintaining their new lower weight lose ½–1 kilogram a week. John's visceral fat score, which gives an indication of cardiovascular disease risk, went from 17 (unhealthy) to 10 (healthy). His slightly high LDL (bad) cholesterol and triglyceride levels returned to a normal range. His blood glucose went from 11.3 (diabetic) to 5.8 (normal). His PSA levels returned to 2.5 – his result when he was 40 years old. When I told him he could modify the rebalance after 28 days, he asked me why he would change something that was working for him! He stopped drinking beer but continued to drink red wine on weekends, although never more than three glasses. His renewed confidence was obvious and he even wore fitted shirts again.

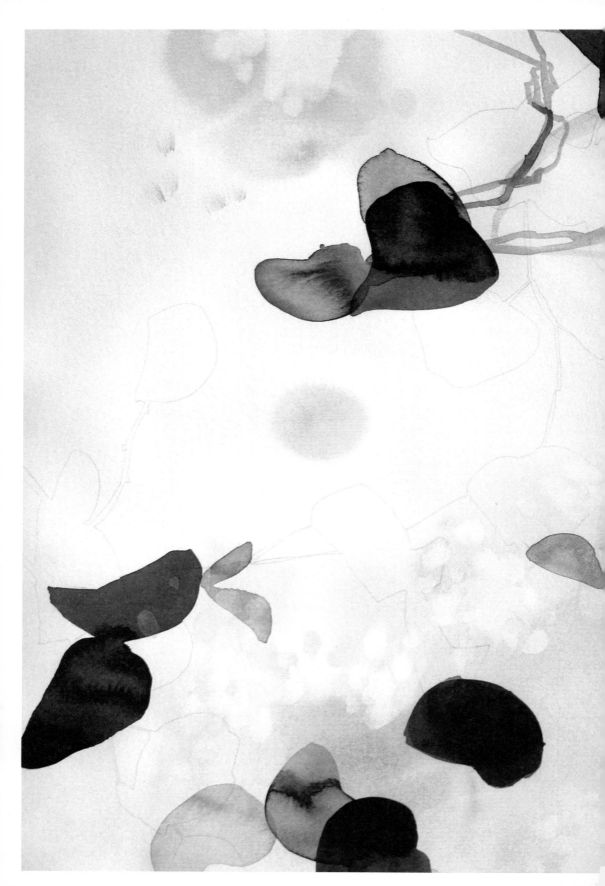

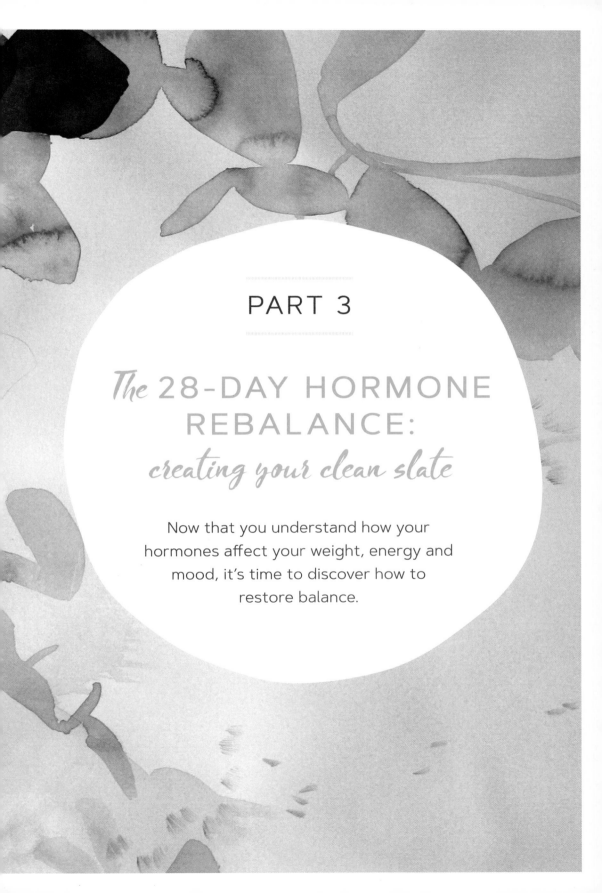

PART 3

The 28-DAY HORMONE REBALANCE:
creating your clean slate

Now that you understand how your hormones affect your weight, energy and mood, it's time to discover how to restore balance.

A WHOLE NEW START

The 28-day Hormone Rebalance gives you the tools and tactics to balance your mood, energy and weight through balancing your hormones. By the end of the plan, you'll be lighter, more vibrant and brimming with energy, and you'll sleep better. I'll outline which foods to put on your plate and explain how different foods affect your delicate hormone balance. It's about creating a new skill set for confidently navigating your way through food choices. I hope this way of eating becomes so easy you don't even need to think about it.

This plan is based on simple principles: to ease digestion and detoxify the liver by eating whole foods. These are foods closest to their natural state and not made in a factory. Whole foods are nutrient-dense carbs, vegetables, easily digestible proteins, low-sugar fruit and good fats free from added sugar, preservatives and additives.

You'll be avoiding foods with added antibiotics, vegetable oils, preservatives and artificial colourings. You'll eliminate foods that are toxin-forming, difficult to digest or cause sensitivities or allergies. I also talk you through the ideal combinations in which to eat food. The aim is to gently eliminate excesses to help your body rejuvenate its filtering system, crank up your metabolism and bring your hormones back into balance.

During the rebalance, I want you to observe how your body reacts to particular foods. You may not be aware of how gluten or dairy affects your body. Once you've removed them from your diet, you can discover if those foods affect how you feel. You'll be 'weeding and seeding'. Weeding removes foods that don't serve you and replaces them with foods that do – that's seeding. I suggest you write down the changes you make to your food and lifestyle and keep track of how you look and feel. Then you can join your own health dots and observe the foods that make you feel good.

It's important to commit fully to the 28 days of the rebalance, as it will set you on a new life path. You'll have more vitality, improved sleep and more energy to play with your children. You'll also be more productive at work and enjoy increased mental clarity.

The first week of the rebalance is relatively easy. By the second and third weeks, you may not love me. But by the fourth week, you'll find it much easier. The gentler you begin, the longer you'll last. One bit of advice: if you fall off the rails, just return to the rebalance at the next meal. Don't beat yourself up. Take a deep breath and get back to it. Smile and be thankful. You cannot fail at good nutrition.

PREPARING FOR THE REBALANCE

Five days before starting the rebalance, begin the weeding process. Your aim is to eliminate — 'crowd out' — red meat, wheat, dairy, sugar, alcohol, caffeine and processed food from your diet. See the following page for more details.

Rather than go cold turkey, each day reduce the amount you eat or drink by half. The next day, decrease the amount by half again. Halve then halve again. I've found that gradually cutting back is more effective than immediate removal. The goal is for lasting, lifelong habits rather than quick weight loss. For example, if you drink two large lattes every day, drop to one large latte and then one regular latte. This isn't the Last Supper, so there's no need to binge before you begin. As the rebalance progresses, some of these foods will be (optionally) reintroduced, including small amounts of alcohol, caffeine and red meat.

During the five-day preparation, it's normal to have headaches or feel tired. Clients who have the greatest success on the rebalance embrace the practice of 'crowding in', or 'seeding'. When you 'crowd in' an abundance of flavoursome, healthy foods, you lose the cravings to eat junk. There's no desire to eat a bread roll or sweet dessert because you're already satisfied.

Take time during your weekend to rest, be quiet, and clean out and restock your pantry, fridge, desk and environment. Withdrawal symptoms vary from person to person. During one cleanse, when I thought my diet and lifestyle were already clean, it felt like I had the flu. Be kind to yourself throughout this process.

PLANNING IS KEY

You're more likely to succeed with the rebalance if you're well prepared. On a practical level, it's about stocking your fridge and pantry with real whole foods (see page 78 for more details). Make a shopping list (see page 80). Do you need to buy a sturdy airtight lunchbox to take meals to the office in?

Is your water bottle convenient to carry and comfortable to drink from? Do you own a teacup that you love using? Have you looked through the recipes, and thought about how to use leftovers (cooking once, but eating twice)? When and how will you take time out to de-stress? Plan, plan, plan.

WEEDING

'Crowd out' the following foods during the rebalance:

* **red meat** – I love to bite into a good burger when I'm back in New York City, but because red meat uses considerable digestive energy, I don't eat it that often. Here's the thing: red meat affects oestrogen levels, and excess oestrogen stops you from getting lean. Red meat is also a probable risk factor in bowel cancer. Plus, when you take a break from eating red meat, there's more space on your plate for vegetables. And the more veggies you eat, the more you'll poo, which is one of the ways oestrogen is excreted. Young vegetarian women have lower oestrogen levels than those who eat meat.

  In this rebalance, grass-fed lamb can be reintroduced in week 3 and other pasture-fed red meat in week 4. I know the cost of buying organic, grass-fed and pasture-fed meat is a barrier for many people. Give it a try during the rebalance and afterwards, buy the very best meat you can afford. One of my strategies is to buy organic or pasture-fed meat when it's on sale and freeze it.

* **milk and most dairy** – On the rebalance you can eat goat's cheese, manchego (a Spanish sheep's cheese) and sheep and goat's yoghurt. By week 3, you can reintroduce plain full-fat Greek yoghurt. I want you to observe your body's reaction from removing dairy. When some people remove dairy, they realise it was the cause of skin irritations, constipation,

a bloated tummy or weight gain. Naturally occurring hormones in some dairy products, including oestrogen and insulin-like growth factor (IGF-1) could have an impact on health, as can antibiotics. I opt for the prevention principle: if there are concerns, avoid it. Drink A2, organic or almond milk.

* **caffeine** – I love drinking coffee but I drink it in moderation. If you have a stressful lifestyle, I'd suggest taking a break from coffee. If you can't quit it entirely, reduce your caffeine hit to one per day. Drink black coffee or replace milk with almond milk. If you can't quit dairy, opt for a little A2 or organic milk. Drink green tea and splurge on herbal teas instead. Dandelion tea is a great substitute for coffee and outstanding at liver cleansing.

  Don't be surprised if you experience a 'caffeine migraine' due to withdrawal. It will only last for a few days. If you're really suffering, drink English breakfast tea or green tea to get you through the preparation period. It's far better to have a little caffeine than pop a paracetamol, because paracetamol affects the liver we're trying to cleanse. Caffeine releases cortisol as part of its fight-or-flight response even if you're just sitting at a desk and, as we've seen, excess cortisol can cause problems with insulin. According to one study, women who consumed four or five cups of coffee per day had 70 per cent more oestrogen than those who drank less than one cup per day. Another study suggests caffeine can lower levels of testosterone, the hormone of vitality, sex and strength.

* **alcohol** – During the rebalance, I'd love you to take a break from all alcohol. If you must indulge in a glass, choose wisely. Drink no more than two standard-sized (100 ml) glasses in one sitting and don't drink for more than two nights during the week. Say no to cocktails and champagne, both of which are full of sugar. Instead, have a moderate-sized glass of red wine or glass of white spirits with soda water and splashes of fresh lemon or lime and mint.

* **sugar** – The withdrawal symptoms from cutting back on sugar could feel worse than the feeling from caffeine withdrawal. Stock your pantry with sweet-tasting teas such as cinnamon, licorice and lemongrass. To calm a craving, add a small pinch of the plant-derived sweetener stevia to your tea. Be assured your body and brain will quickly adapt to eating savoury foods, and you'll enjoy renewed energy and mental clarity from cutting out the white stuff. Another way to dampen sugar cravings is to add quality fats, such as fish oil supplements, flaxseeds or avocados. Eat sweet potatoes and pumpkin to satisfy your sweet tastebuds, or have some yoghurt with cinnamon or vanilla bean extract.

* **bread, pasta or wheat products** – Please don't immediately close this book and run to a bakery! I have Italian heritage and understand the appeal of bread, pasta and foods that contain gluten, including wheat, rye, barley and oats. During the rebalance, you're creating a clean slate, so gluten is off the menu to enable you to find out how your body feels when it's removed. If you find you don't react to gluten, you can return it to your meals. But you may find you feel much better. In this way, I want you to join your health dots. During the plan, you'll be eating quality proteins, good fats such as avocado and olive oil, and sweet-tasting slow-release carbs such as pumpkin and sweet potato. You won't even miss the bread that could have made you puffy, bloated and brain-fogged.

* **processed foods** – If it's been made in a factory and is full of chemicals that don't occur naturally in foods, throw it out. After the rebalance you can go back to eating 'clean' grab-and-go foods, but for the next 28 days, choose real, whole foods.

You'll crowd in so much yummy food that you'll forget the junk food of your past. This plan is about nourishment, not deprivation. You should never feel hungry during the rebalance.

SEEDING

'Crowd in' the following during the rebalance (see the following pages for a complete shopping list)

* **veggies** – Packed with antioxidants, and fibre that makes you feel full. Green leafy vegetables and cruciferous veggies such as cauliflower, broccoli, kale, cabbage and turnip help your liver detoxify.
* **healthy fats** – Avocado, seeds, nuts, coconut oil, olive oil, salmon and trout.
* **protein foods** – Chicken, fish, eggs, non-dairy cheese and yoghurt, seeds and nuts, which stabilise blood sugar levels and make you feel satisfied.
* **fibre** – Try flaxseeds, chia seeds and fibrous vegetables, which cleanse the bowel and lower LDL cholesterol. Fibre helps control weight.
* **water, herbal teas and sparkling water** – Some people confuse hunger with thirst. Keep hydrated. Drink six to eight glasses of filtered water a day. Drink up to three cups of green tea a day. Even though it contains a small amount of caffeine, green tea is high in antioxidants. Decaffeinated green tea is also available.
* **daily exercise** – Try taking a walk in the sunshine or doing high-intensity interval training (HIIT), a short burst of intense activity followed by a short period of recovery. The original HIIT formula was 20 seconds of intensity at 80 per cent of your maximum heart rate, followed by 12 seconds of rest over the course of 20 minutes. Another option is 45 seconds of intensity followed by 15 seconds of rest over 30 minutes. This method improves insulin resistance and weight loss. Use your judgement: for the first five days, be gentle with yourself. If you feel tired, exhausted or headachy, don't worry. These are normal signs of detoxification. Go to bed early or take a bath in magnesium-rich and calming Epsom salts.
* **sleep** – During the rebalance, sleep for a minimum of eight hours per night to assist hormone regulation, improved levels of neurotransmitters and boosted immunity. The healthy people I know are very protective of their sleep, exercise and nutrition, and they don't compromise or make excuses. Remind yourself that the rebalance is for a time and place, not forever, and is a foundation for sustainable weight loss, balanced moods and vibrant energy.

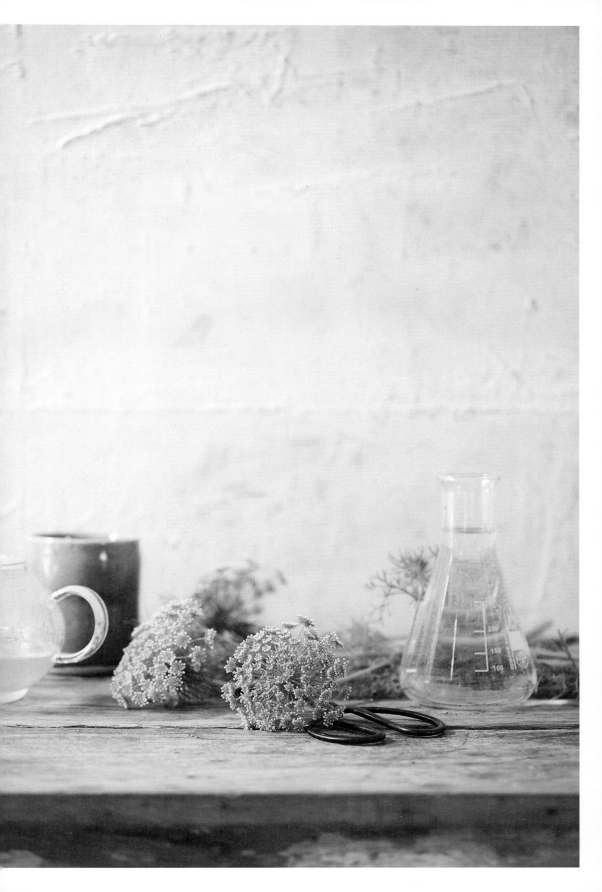

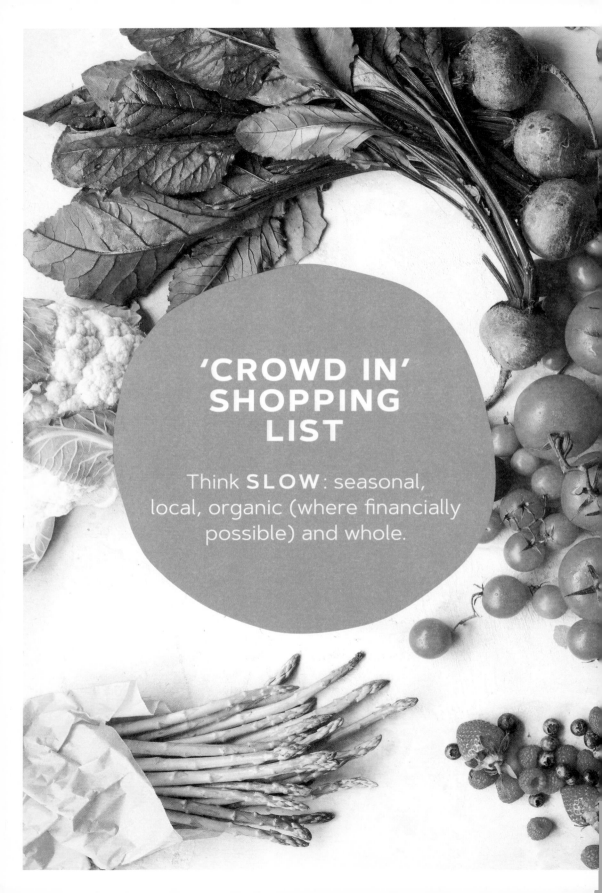

'CROWD IN' SHOPPING LIST

Think **SLOW**: seasonal, local, organic (where financially possible) and whole.

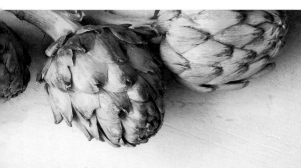

FRUIT

* Apples
* Berries – blueberries, raspberries and strawberries (fresh or frozen)
* Grapefruit
* Kiwi fruit
* Lemon and lime – for teas and water
* Pears

STARCHY VEGETABLES

If your goal is to lose weight, limit starchy vegetables to once a day at breakfast or lunch. Starchy veggies are a great substitute for bread and an outstanding fuel source. My favourite is the baked sweet potato that features daily in my meals or snacks.

* Artichokes
* Beetroot
* Carrots
* Celeriac
* Corn
* Edamame (fresh or frozen)
* Parsnip
* Potatoes
* Pumpkin
* Sweet potatoes
* Yams

NON-STARCHY AND LOW-STARCH VEGETABLES

* Asparagus
* Avocado (sometimes classed as a fruit but I think of it as a veggie)
* Bok choy
* Broccoli*
* Brussels sprouts*
* Cabbage*
* Capsicum
* Cauliflower*
* Celery
* Cucumber
* Dandelion greens
* Eggplant
* Fennel
* Green beans
* Kale*
* Leek
* Lettuce
* Olives
* Onion
* Peas
* Pickled or fermented vegetables
* Radish
* Rocket
* Shiitake mushrooms
* Spinach
* Sprouts
* Tomatoes
* Turnip
* Watercress

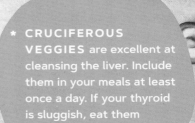

* **CRUCIFEROUS VEGGIES** are excellent at cleansing the liver. Include them in your meals at least once a day. If your thyroid is sluggish, eat them cooked rather than raw.

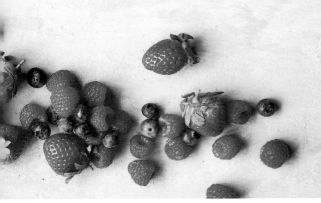

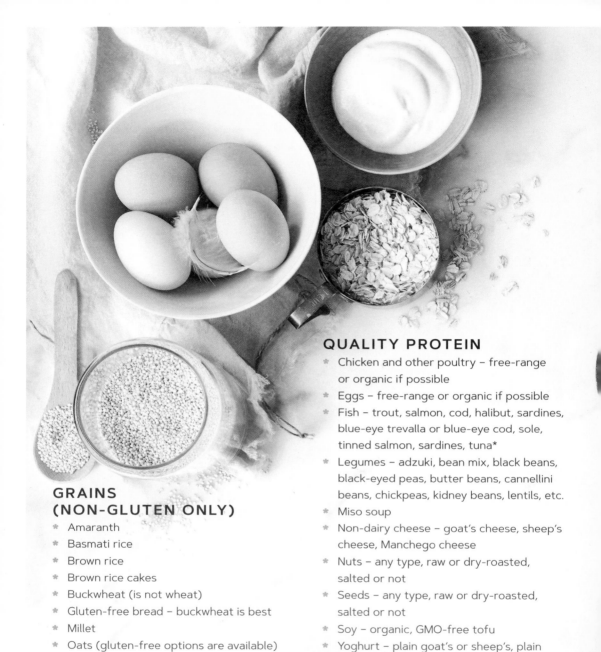

GRAINS (NON-GLUTEN ONLY)

* Amaranth
* Basmati rice
* Brown rice
* Brown rice cakes
* Buckwheat (is not wheat)
* Gluten-free bread – buckwheat is best
* Millet
* Oats (gluten-free options are available)
* Quinoa

QUALITY PROTEIN

* Chicken and other poultry – free-range or organic if possible
* Eggs – free-range or organic if possible
* Fish – trout, salmon, cod, halibut, sardines, blue-eye trevalla or blue-eye cod, sole, tinned salmon, sardines, tuna*
* Legumes – adzuki, bean mix, black beans, black-eyed peas, butter beans, cannellini beans, chickpeas, kidney beans, lentils, etc.
* Miso soup
* Non-dairy cheese – goat's cheese, sheep's cheese, Manchego cheese
* Nuts – any type, raw or dry-roasted, salted or not
* Seeds – any type, raw or dry-roasted, salted or not
* Soy – organic, GMO-free tofu
* Yoghurt – plain goat's or sheep's, plain Greek yoghurt (from week 3)

* Because of its mercury content, eat no more than two tins of tuna a week.

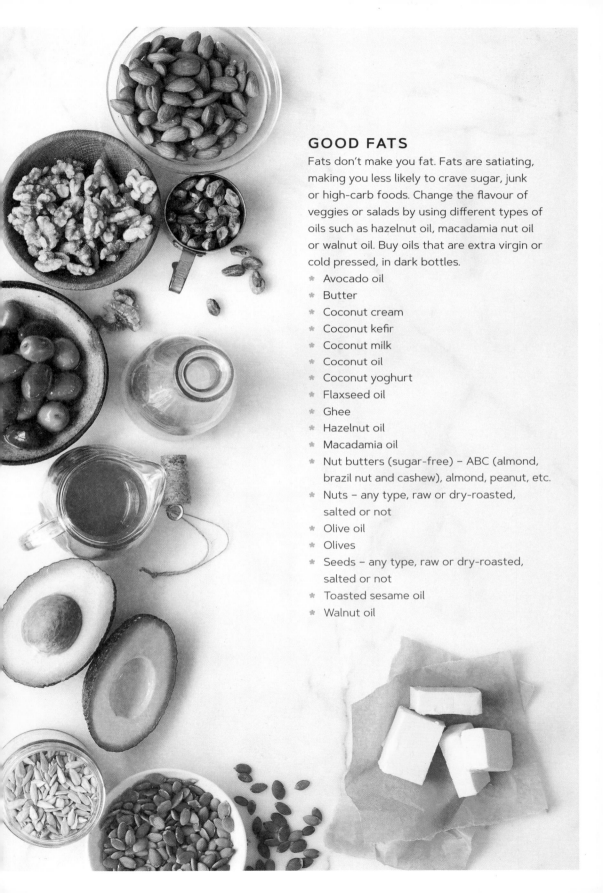

GOOD FATS

Fats don't make you fat. Fats are satiating, making you less likely to crave sugar, junk or high-carb foods. Change the flavour of veggies or salads by using different types of oils such as hazelnut oil, macadamia nut oil or walnut oil. Buy oils that are extra virgin or cold pressed, in dark bottles.

* Avocado oil
* Butter
* Coconut cream
* Coconut kefir
* Coconut milk
* Coconut oil
* Coconut yoghurt
* Flaxseed oil
* Ghee
* Hazelnut oil
* Macadamia oil
* Nut butters (sugar-free) – ABC (almond, brazil nut and cashew), almond, peanut, etc.
* Nuts – any type, raw or dry-roasted, salted or not
* Olive oil
* Olives
* Seeds – any type, raw or dry-roasted, salted or not
* Toasted sesame oil
* Walnut oil

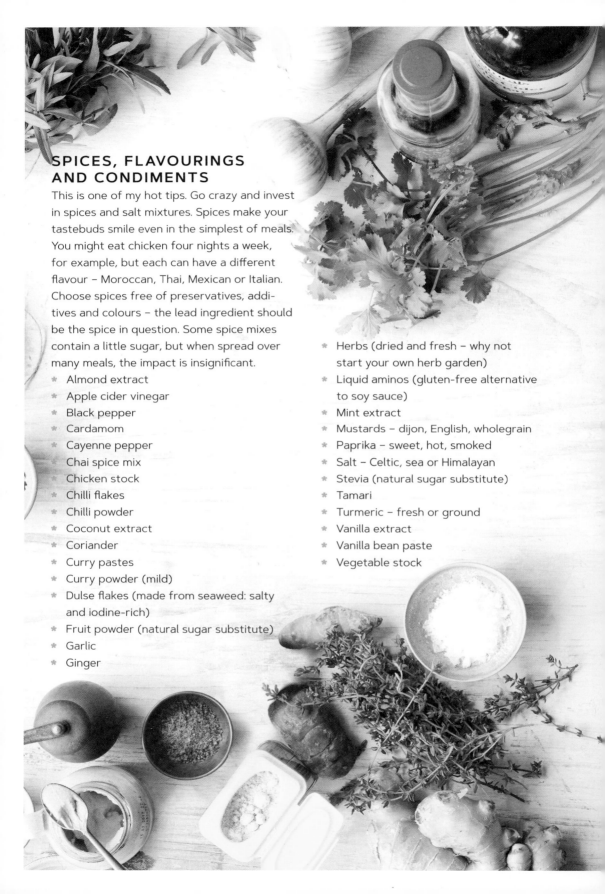

SPICES, FLAVOURINGS AND CONDIMENTS

This is one of my hot tips. Go crazy and invest in spices and salt mixtures. Spices make your tastebuds smile even in the simplest of meals. You might eat chicken four nights a week, for example, but each can have a different flavour – Moroccan, Thai, Mexican or Italian. Choose spices free of preservatives, additives and colours – the lead ingredient should be the spice in question. Some spice mixes contain a little sugar, but when spread over many meals, the impact is insignificant.

* Almond extract
* Apple cider vinegar
* Black pepper
* Cardamom
* Cayenne pepper
* Chai spice mix
* Chicken stock
* Chilli flakes
* Chilli powder
* Coconut extract
* Coriander
* Curry pastes
* Curry powder (mild)
* Dulse flakes (made from seaweed: salty and iodine-rich)
* Fruit powder (natural sugar substitute)
* Garlic
* Ginger
* Herbs (dried and fresh – why not start your own herb garden)
* Liquid aminos (gluten-free alternative to soy sauce)
* Mint extract
* Mustards – dijon, English, wholegrain
* Paprika – sweet, hot, smoked
* Salt – Celtic, sea or Himalayan
* Stevia (natural sugar substitute)
* Tamari
* Turmeric – fresh or ground
* Vanilla extract
* Vanilla bean paste
* Vegetable stock

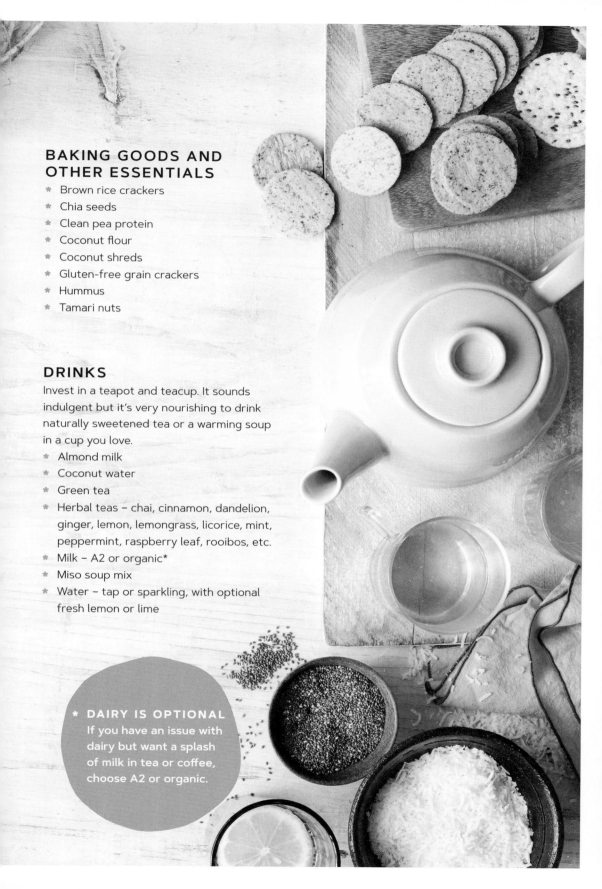

BAKING GOODS AND OTHER ESSENTIALS

* Brown rice crackers
* Chia seeds
* Clean pea protein
* Coconut flour
* Coconut shreds
* Gluten-free grain crackers
* Hummus
* Tamari nuts

DRINKS

Invest in a teapot and teacup. It sounds indulgent but it's very nourishing to drink naturally sweetened tea or a warming soup in a cup you love.

* Almond milk
* Coconut water
* Green tea
* Herbal teas – chai, cinnamon, dandelion, ginger, lemon, lemongrass, licorice, mint, peppermint, raspberry leaf, rooibos, etc.
* Milk – A2 or organic*
* Miso soup mix
* Water – tap or sparkling, with optional fresh lemon or lime

* DAIRY IS OPTIONAL
If you have an issue with dairy but want a splash of milk in tea or coffee, choose A2 or organic.

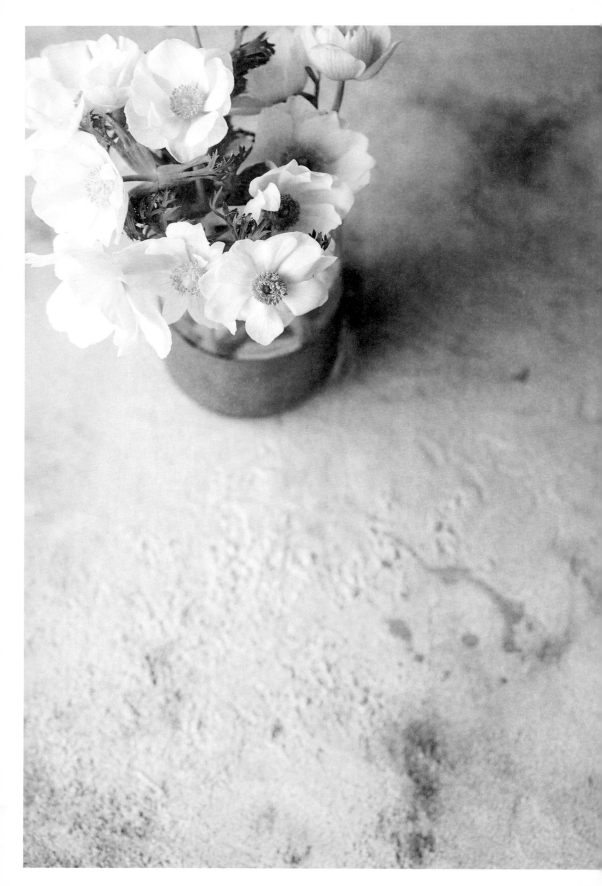

THE REBALANCE EXPLAINED

During the rebalance, you'll be eating three meals and two snacks each day. Don't skip any meals or snacks in the first week. This will cause your blood sugar levels to drop and you want to keep these as stable as possible to maintain energy, satiation and an even hormone keel. You shouldn't feel hungry at all on this program.

Breakfasts and lunches will be simple combinations of whole foods – see the meal suggestions on pages 92–95. (And for lunches, leftovers from dinner the night before are also a great option.)

For dinner, I've provided you with a daily recipe that incorporates the changing requirements each week. You can swap these around within the week, but not between weeks. Or you can use the food-combining rules along with the simple steps on the following page to create your own meals.

THE 28-DAY HORMONE REBALANCE **AT A GLANCE**

	Crowd out	Crowd in	Additional changes
Week 1	Red meat, wheat, dairy, sugar, alcohol, caffeine and processed food.	Veggies, healthy fats, white meat, non-dairy cheese and yoghurt, eggs, fibre, water, herbal teas and sparkling water, daily exercise and rest.	-
Week 2	As week 1.	As week 1.	From day 14, try intermittent fasting by skipping one dinner (no more) during the week.
Week 3	Red meat (apart from grass-fed lamb), wheat, dairy, sugar, alcohol, caffeine and processed food.	As weeks 1 and 2, but you can reintroduce grass-fed lamb, unless you feel better without it.	Continue intermittent fasting, skipping one dinner during the week.
Week 4	Wheat, dairy, sugar, alcohol, caffeine and processed food.	As week 3, but you can reintroduce grass-fed red meat. As there's only one more week left, hold off if you can.	-

FIVE FOOD-COMBINING
RULES FOR A CLEAN SLATE

I've successfully used food-combining principles with clients since 2005. It works to maximise digestion based on the theory that we digest different foods at different speeds. After applying these rules, most of my clients tell me they didn't even realise they felt sluggish until their energy came bursting back. When you follow these rules, you enhance gut health, improve digestion and reduce gas and bloating. When digestion is lighter, your body can absorb rich nutrients such as vitamins, minerals and antioxidants.

1. ONLY EAT GRAINS WITH VEGETABLES

You can combine starchy and non-starchy vegetables from the shopping list on page 81. If your goal is to lose weight, eat starchy vegetables no more than once a day at breakfast or lunch. Vegetables should take up more than 50 per cent of your plate. This doesn't mean that eating fish (a protein) and rice (a grain) in the same meal is bad for you, but during the rebalance, you want to lighten the digestive burden. Grains take two to three hours to digest. I suggest eating grains for breakfast or lunch because slow, smart carbs fuel the brain and muscles when needed – during the day rather than in the evening. Grains are a great source of fibre and so help keep the bowels moving.

2. ONLY EAT PROTEINS WITH VEGETABLES

Protein is the most complex nutrient to digest, taking two to six hours to process. Add an abundance of low-starch and starchy veggies to proteins. Remember: this plan is not about starving yourself. Protein and veggies are the ideal combination for dinner because you don't need energy from carbs during sleep.

3. DON'T EAT PROTEINS AND GRAINS IN THE SAME MEAL

Non-gluten grains and protein need energy for digestion. I want that energy focused on toxin elimination and cellular renewal. You'll eat starchy veggies (root veggies) and a ton of non-starchy veggies (green leafy veggies). When not following the rebalance program, it's not wrong to eat fish and rice or chicken and quinoa together, but if you do, you'll expend more energy digesting it.

4. EAT ONE PROTEIN FOOD PER MEAL

The simpler the meal, the easier it is to digest. If preparing an omelette for breakfast, add mushrooms or sautéed vegetables rather than cheese. Include leftover vegetables from last night's meal. Double the amount of veggies you place in the baking tray – cook once, eat twice.

5. EAT FRUIT ON ITS OWN

Yes, that's right. If you like to eat fruit and yoghurt at the same time, then sorry. Sugars in fruit are digested quickly – in around 20 minutes to one hour. Protein takes longer to digest. When protein and sugar land in the stomach at the same time, digestion is more complicated and can cause a sore stomach. When some people eat fruit after muesli or eggs, they get a puffy tummy. If you feel bloated or gassy, this tip alone could turn your tummy around. During the rebalance, eat low-sugar fruits such as apples, pears, grapefruit, kiwi fruit or berries. To keep the rules simple, only eat fruit at morning or afternoon tea and one hour either side of meals. Remember, the rebalance is not forever – it's an opportunity for you to discover what works best for you.

SIMPLE STEPS FOR CONSTRUCTING A MEAL

Step 1   Select a protein or grain
Step 2   Select several veggies
Step 3   Create a spice mix
Step 4   Choose a quality fat
Step 5   Make a dressing or marinade (see pages 216–17).

FOOD COMBINING RULES FOR A CLEAN SLATE

QUALITY PROTEIN

GOOD FATS

FRUIT

VEGETABLES

NON-GLUTEN GRAINS

BEFORE BREAKFAST DRINKS

Kickstart your day with some of these balancing pre-brekkie drinks.

fresh vegetable juice with lemon and ginger perfect for those warmer months

rooibos tea
perfect all year round

warm water with lemon
perfect all year round

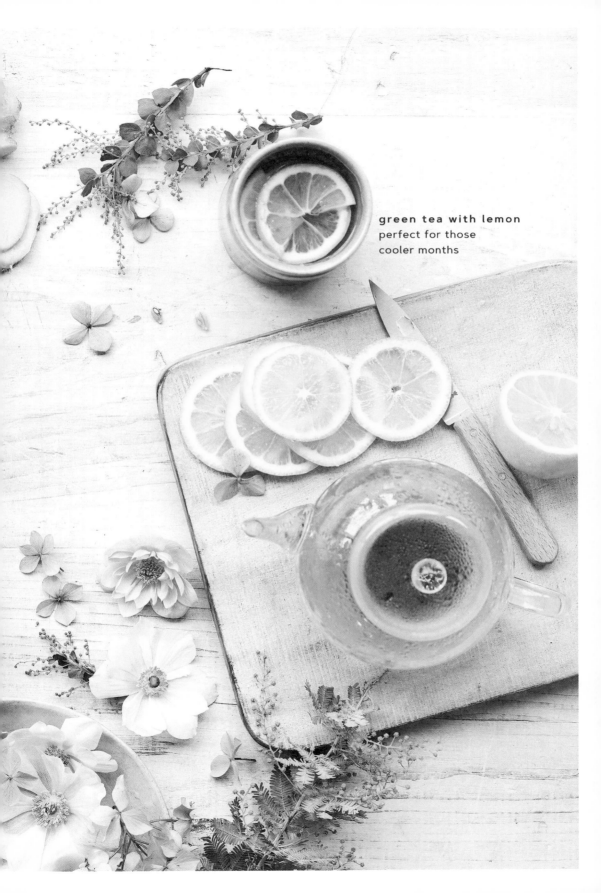

green tea with lemon
perfect for those
cooler months

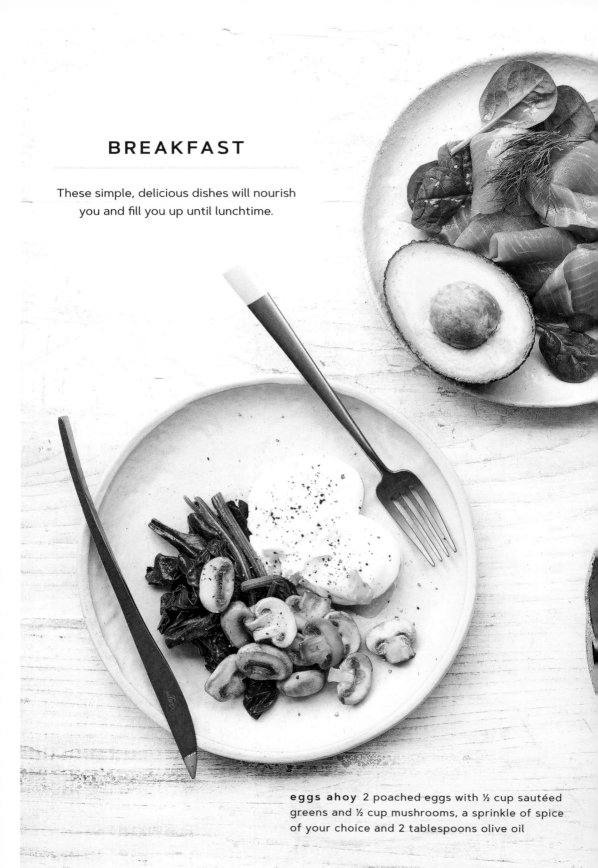

BREAKFAST

These simple, delicious dishes will nourish
you and fill you up until lunchtime.

eggs ahoy 2 poached eggs with ½ cup sautéed
greens and ½ cup mushrooms, a sprinkle of spice
of your choice and 2 tablespoons olive oil

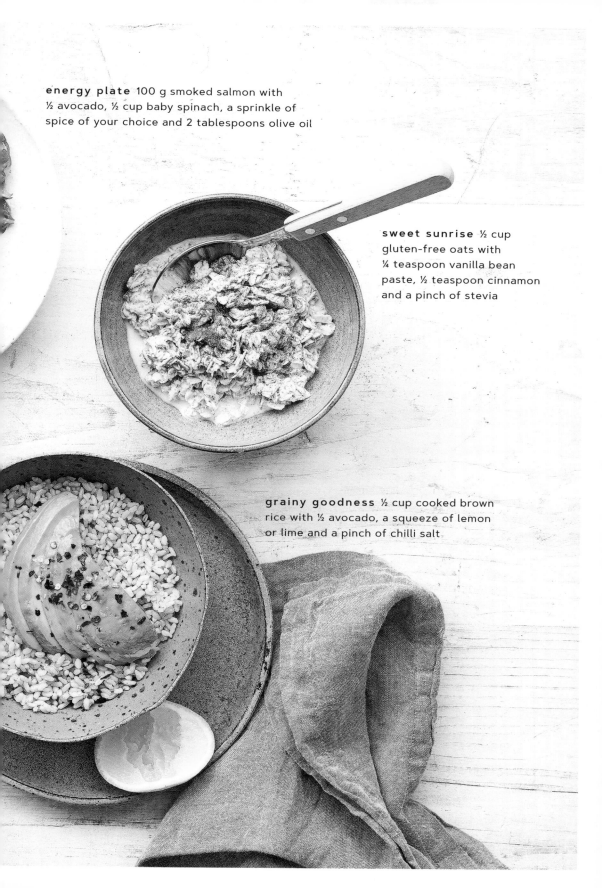

energy plate 100 g smoked salmon with ½ avocado, ½ cup baby spinach, a sprinkle of spice of your choice and 2 tablespoons olive oil

sweet sunrise ½ cup gluten-free oats with ¼ teaspoon vanilla bean paste, ½ teaspoon cinnamon and a pinch of stevia

grainy goodness ½ cup cooked brown rice with ½ avocado, a squeeze of lemon or lime and a pinch of chilli salt

LUNCH

Here are some ideas that can be cooked on the spot or prepared in advance to make your life easier. Also, remember the simplest lunch is leftovers from last night's dinner – cook once, eat twice!

brown rice bowl ½ cup cooked brown rice, 1 cup cooked veggies, a pinch of your favourite spice mix, a squeeze of lemon juice, 2 tablespoons walnut oil, top with chopped herbs or chilli

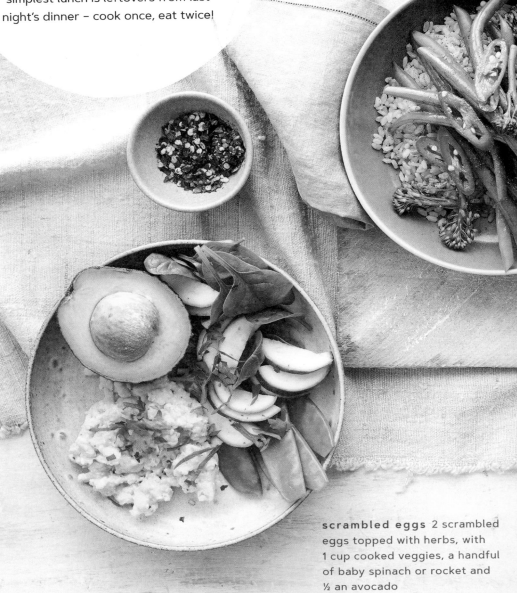

scrambled eggs 2 scrambled eggs topped with herbs, with 1 cup cooked veggies, a handful of baby spinach or rocket and ½ an avocado

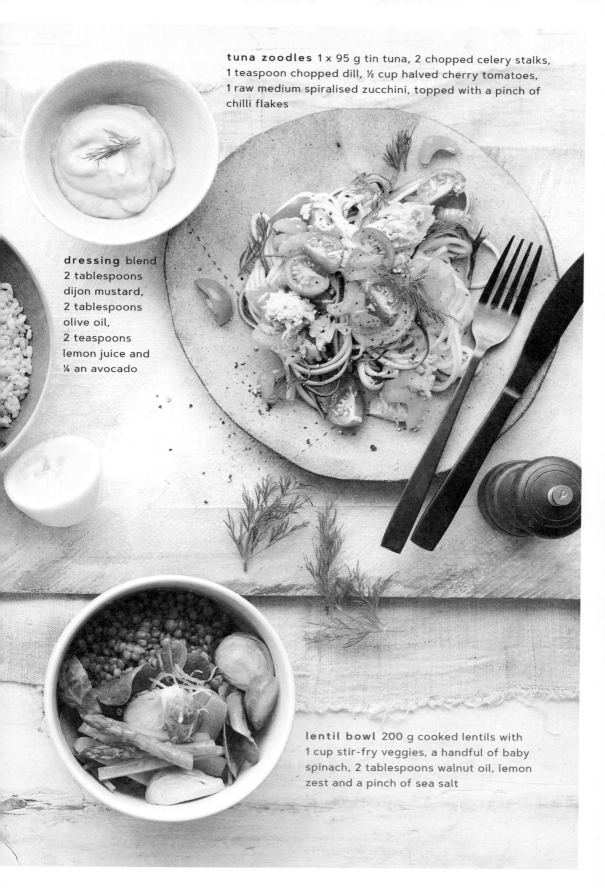

tuna zoodles 1 x 95 g tin tuna, 2 chopped celery stalks, 1 teaspoon chopped dill, ½ cup halved cherry tomatoes, 1 raw medium spiralised zucchini, topped with a pinch of chilli flakes

dressing blend 2 tablespoons dijon mustard, 2 tablespoons olive oil, 2 teaspoons lemon juice and ¼ an avocado

lentil bowl 200 g cooked lentils with 1 cup stir-fry veggies, a handful of baby spinach, 2 tablespoons walnut oil, lemon zest and a pinch of sea salt

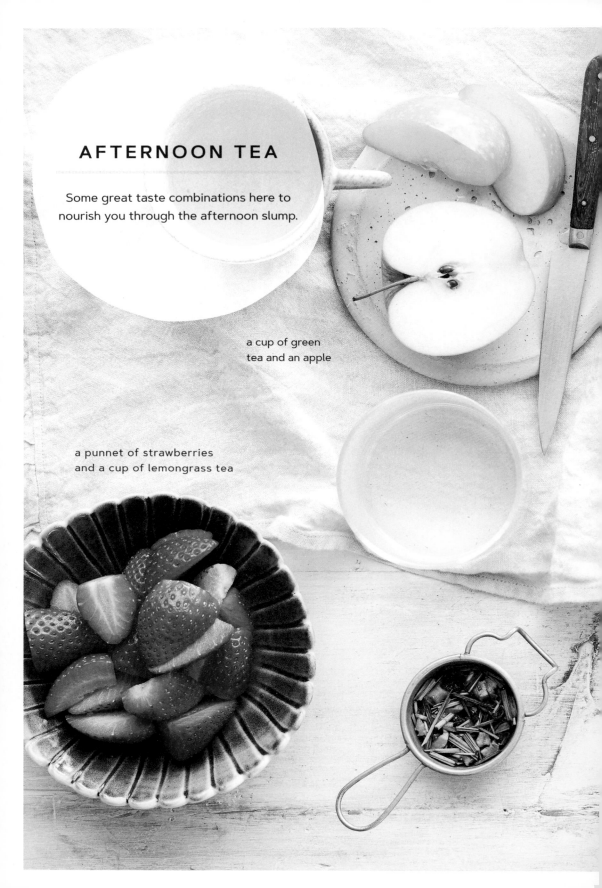

AFTERNOON TEA

Some great taste combinations here to nourish you through the afternoon slump.

a cup of green
tea and an apple

a punnet of strawberries
and a cup of lemongrass tea

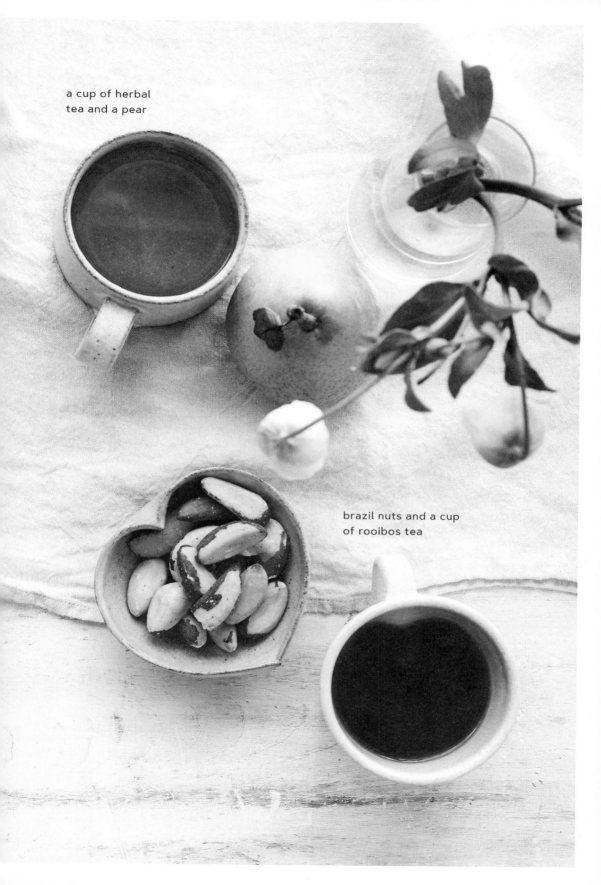

a cup of herbal
tea and a pear

brazil nuts and a cup
of rooibos tea

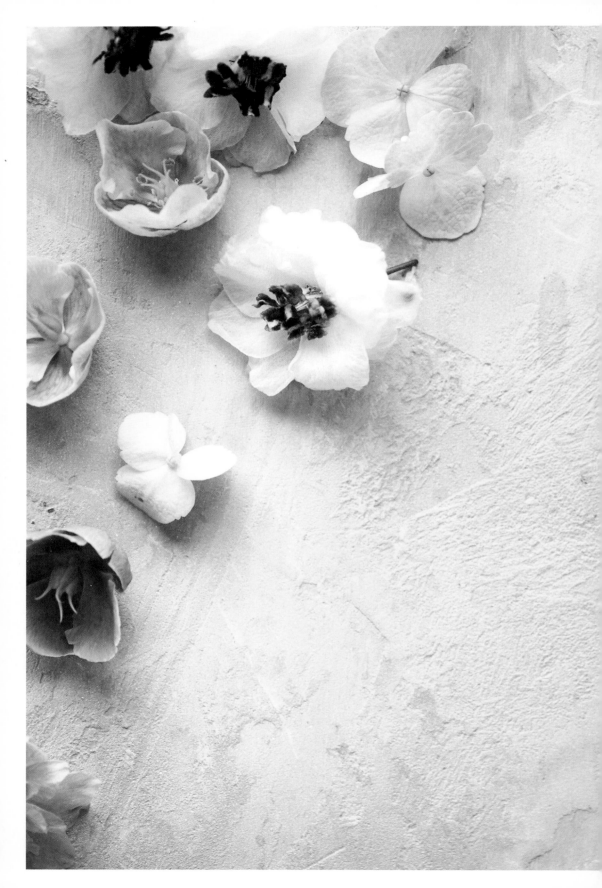

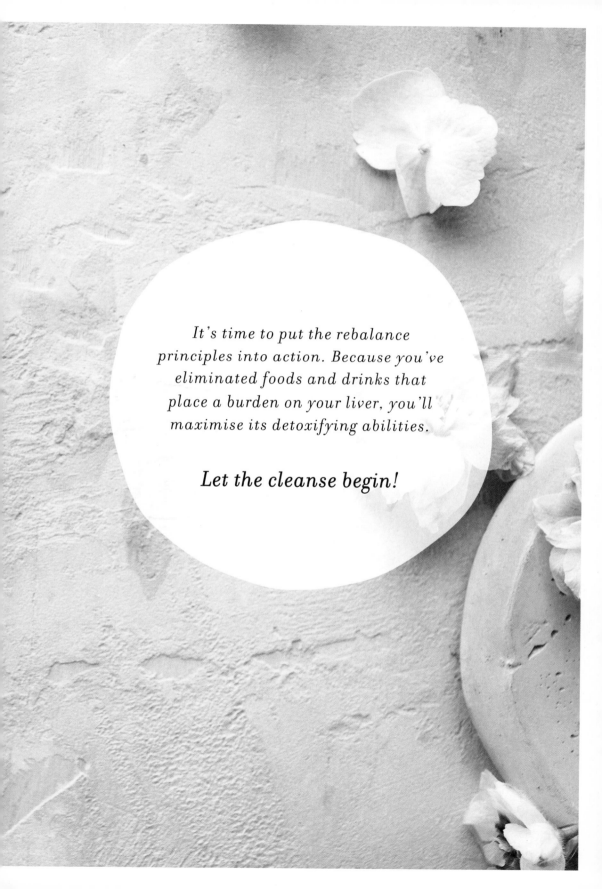

It's time to put the rebalance principles into action. Because you've eliminated foods and drinks that place a burden on your liver, you'll maximise its detoxifying abilities.

Let the cleanse begin!

DAY 1

Make the **hormone rebalance** a priority

I'm not going to sugar-coat this for you. The habits you've formed over your lifetime will be challenging to break. That's why I need you to make a commitment to this rebalance for the next 28 days. If you want to look and feel healthy, improve your sleep and balance your moods, this must be the priority in your life.

You need to set aside time for meal preparation. And you need to get strategic when faced with food choices away from home. Each evening, make a food plan for the following day and write it down, ensuring it adheres to the principles. Follow the daily recipes. Choose high-quality proteins, good fats and complex carbohydrates. The aim is to keep your blood sugar steady so you don't become ravenous. When we become ravenous and haven't prepared for the next meal or snack, we often overeat. When we overeat, excess insulin sends a message to fat cells to absorb excess glucose and turn it into fat.

Did you recognise yourself in one of the case studies described earlier in the book? Did you have a light-bulb moment? You know the time to make changes to your nutrition and lifestyle is now. As you begin a journey of nourishment, not deprivation, take a deep, slow, smiling breath. This sustainable 28-day plan will become an invaluable tool you can apply beyond the rebalance. I promise you will not starve. I was a yo-yo dieter until I learned, understood and embraced the rebalance plan and you can do this too.

One way to keep motivated with the plan is to set incentives and rewards. For example, write down the reward you'll give yourself if you diligently follow the program for 28 days. It could be a new item of clothing, a meal out or an experience. That way, when your willpower is challenged, you can project your mind forward to the reward as a way of keeping on track. And remember: it's only 28 days.

TODAY'S ACTION

Today, I want you to clearly define your goal. Do you want more energy, improved mood, better-quality sleep or to lose the muffin top or man boobs? Go on. Do it now. Write down your goal. When faced with temptation, such as a slice of cake for a colleague's birthday – even a sliver of a slice – this goal will propel you to make the decision that best serves you. If you happen to go off the rails at one meal, or for one night, don't beat yourself up. Let it go. And don't use the derailment and feelings of guilt as an excuse to blow the remainder of your day. Guilt plays a significant role in emotional eating. Don't go there. Acknowledge the blip and return to the rebalance.

CHARGRILLED SALMON WITH CORIANDER SALSA

Salmon is a nutritional star, packed with essential fatty acids and omega-3 fats.
Quality fat is excellent for the brain and our sex hormones.

PREPARATION TIME: 10 MINUTES, PLUS STANDING TIME
COOKING TIME: 20 MINUTES ♥ SERVES 4

4 × 150 g wild-caught
    salmon fillets, skin on,
    bones removed
1 tablespoon extra virgin
    olive oil
pinch of sea salt
pinch of freshly ground
    black pepper
lemon or lime wedges, to serve

CORIANDER SALSA
1 tablespoon extra virgin
    olive oil
1 small bunch coriander,
    leaves picked
2 tablespoons chopped mint
2 tablespoons finely
    chopped garlic
1 tablespoon finely grated
    lemon or lime zest
1 tablespoon lemon or
    lime juice
pinch of chilli flakes (optional)

Coat the salmon in the olive oil and season with the salt and pepper. Set aside for 10 minutes.

To make the salsa, combine all the ingredients in a blender and blend until smooth and fragrant. Set aside.

Heat a chargrill pan or barbecue grill plate over medium–high heat. Place the fish, skin-side down, on the grill and cook for about 15 minutes or until the skin is charred and the fish is almost cooked through. Turn over and grill for a few more minutes, until the fish is fully cooked. Remove from the heat and place the salmon, skin-side up, on a plate. Remove the skin, then turn the salmon over and spoon the salsa over the top. Serve with lemon or lime wedges.

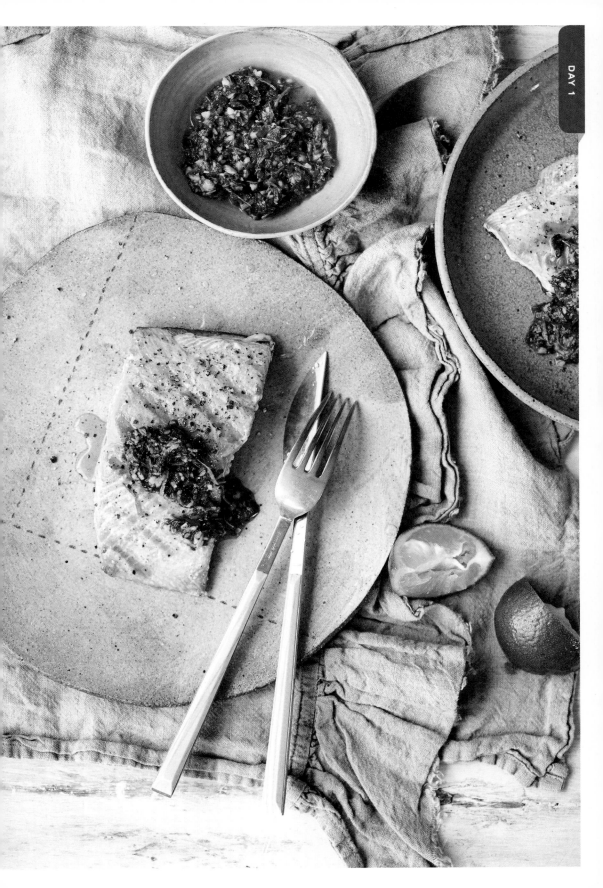

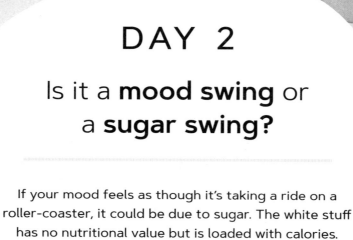

DAY 2

Is it a **mood swing** or a **sugar swing?**

If your mood feels as though it's taking a ride on a roller-coaster, it could be due to sugar. The white stuff has no nutritional value but is loaded with calories. Every time you consume sugar you feel an initial rush, but it's fleeting, and sugar lacks the vitamins and minerals your body needs to function. And here's the thing: when you eat processed foods laced with hidden sugars, there's not enough room in your stomach for protein-rich, fibre-filled foods.

Protein supports the immune system and creates lean muscle mass. It breaks down to an amino acid called tryptophan. One way the body makes serotonin is to combine tryptophan with B vitamins. If you eat sugary, poor-quality carbs, you don't ingest adequate tryptophan or B vitamins. Plus, if you consume too much sugar you feel good in the short term from the release of dopamine. But as with any addictive drug, your system can become desensitised to the dopamine released, needing more and more each time to experience the same pleasure.

In order to break an addiction to sugar, find out where the sweet stuff lurks. Hidden sugar is everywhere, so you need to become what I call a 'label detective'. Look for the sugar pseudonyms on food labels, including fructose, lactose, maltose, agave and barley malt (see the full list on page 219).

And then there's the task of working out how many teaspoons of sugar is in the food. On the label, find the total sugar per serving in grams and divide that number by four. This is the approximate number of teaspoons of sugar in the serving (and bear in mind that the World Health Organization recommends no more than 6 teaspoons of sugar a day). This method isn't exact, and doesn't take into account natural sugars, but it's a good general indicator of hidden sugar.

TODAY'S ACTION

Today your focus is on your sugar intake. Limit consumption to natural sources from low-sugar fruits and vegetables. After the rebalance, you shouldn't consume processed foods that contain more than 5 grams of sugar per 100 grams. (Remember, eating two slices of some brands of wholegrain bread can add more than 2 tablespoons of sugar.) If you need a sweet hit, drink cinnamon tea or licorice tea.

FINDING HIDDEN SUGARS

The sugars hidden in packaged and prepared foods include table sugar (sucrose), high-fructose corn syrup, honey, syrups, fruit juices and fruit concentrate. Because they're hidden, they're health hijackers. When fruit is in juice form, it comes minus the fibre and has the same effect on blood sugar as drinking cola. Yes, apple juice contains some vitamins so it's not all bad, but foods with fibre blunt the blood sugar spike. A small bottle of apple juice can contain the juice from five apples. Would you ever eat five apples in one sitting? When fruits are juiced, their fibre is removed and we're left with a cup of concentrated sugar. There's more joy in crunching into an apple than gulping down a juice.

WARM BRUSSELS SPROUTS CHICKEN CAESAR SALAD

Brussels sprouts are part of the brassica (also known as cruciferous) family, and have a cleansing effect on the liver. Happy hormones love a naturally detoxed liver.

PREPARATION TIME: 15 MINUTES, PLUS MARINATING TIME
COOKING TIME: 30 MINUTES ♥ SERVES 4

4 x 150 g skinless chicken
   breast fillets
1 tablespoon extra virgin
   olive oil
500 g brussels sprouts,
   thinly sliced
chopped flat-leaf parsley,
   to garnish

DRESSING
½ cup extra virgin olive oil
1 teaspoon finely grated
   lemon zest
⅓ cup lemon juice
2 garlic cloves,
   roughly chopped
3 teaspoons dijon mustard
2 teaspoons tamari
2 teaspoons capers, rinsed
sea salt and freshly ground
   black pepper (optional)

To make the dressing, combine the olive oil, lemon zest, lemon juice, garlic, mustard, tamari and capers in a blender and blend until smooth. Taste and season if required.

Place the chicken in a glass or ceramic dish, then pour half the dressing evenly over the top. Set aside to marinate for at least 15 minutes (though if you can, prepare this in the morning or even the night before so it has plenty of time to marinate). The dressing will keep for up to 3 days in the refrigerator.

Preheat the oven to 180°C.

Transfer the chicken breasts to a baking dish and bake for 20–25 minutes or until cooked through. Alternatively, cook them on the barbecue.

Meanwhile, heat the olive oil in a frying pan over medium heat, add the sprouts and sauté for about 5 minutes or until just tender. Transfer to a large bowl.

Toss the remaining dressing through the sprouts. Slice the chicken and scatter over the top, then garnish with flat-leaf parsley and serve.

TIP: *If brussels sprouts aren't your thing, use 1 head of romaine lettuce, roughly chopped, instead. Just toss it with the dressing and serve with the chicken and parsley.*

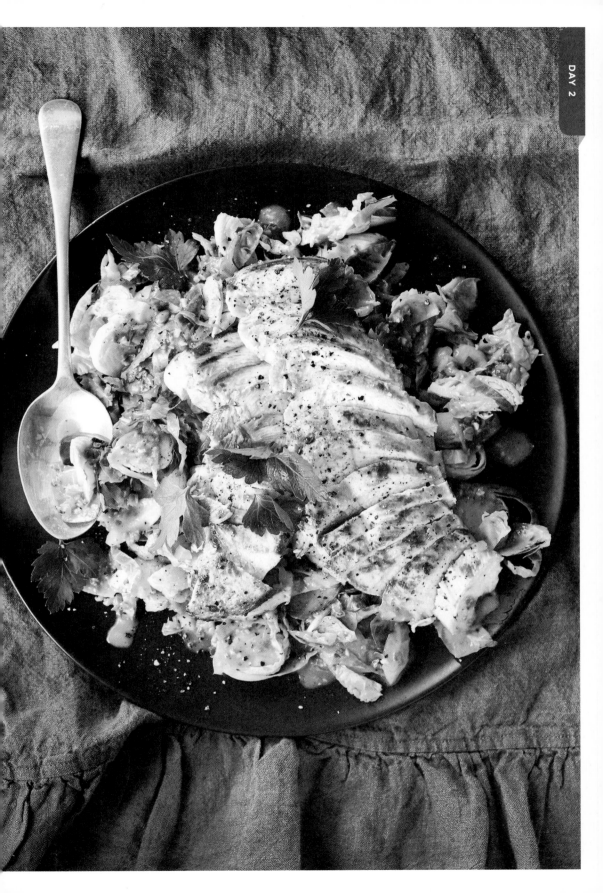

DAY 3

Portion **distortion**

Discussing portion sizes can be tricky, because I believe that weighing and measuring food removes some of the joy from eating it. Eating should be about sharing with family and friends. Let's bring back the love of food. Let's stop counting calories and behaving like the 'food police'. On this plan, you'll be pleasantly surprised at how much you can eat. Why? Because eating clean, whole, real food sends a signal to your brain to indicate when you are full. You simply won't have room for the junky, sugary stuff of the past.

When I was juggling the demands of three young children, work, laundry and life, I would 'stress eat'. Most of us do. Instead of listening to the signals that I was satisfied, I ate to excess even though I was full. After my babies went to bed, I became a human vacuum cleaner. Instead of eating one apple with nut butter, I would have two with half a jar of nut butter. I had the 'portion distortion' that often comes with stress and lack of sleep. I still have bouts of emotional eating, but when it comes on I stop and ask myself if I'm feeling tired. Eating six handfuls of nuts in one sitting won't fix things, but maybe an early night will.

Portion sizes have slowly but surely increased to the extent that we now believe that larger servings are standard. And because we're trained to finish eating everything on our plates, it means we're consuming more calories than we need to. (At some fast-food outlets, you can consume your entire daily calories in one meal!) At first, it's difficult to leave food on your plate. It feels wrong. But training yourself to be conscious about food portions will get you to your ultimate goal of balanced and healthy eating.

Even if we eat good-quality food, we can eat too much of it and put on weight. The switch to smart low-carb, low-sugar foods in the rebalance will make you feel more satisfied even as you keep your portions under control.

TODAY'S ACTION

It's not practical to carry around a set of scales and weigh everything before you eat it. You could use scales initially to get a sense of portion size. Then use your hands, consulting the table on page 218.

ROASTED CARROT SOUP
WITH THAI FLAVOURS

I love Thai flavours, particularly with carrots. Carrots are rich in phytonutrient antioxidants such as beta-carotene and vitamin C. Feel free to swap the carrot with other root vegetables.

PREPARATION TIME: 15 MINUTES ♥ COOKING TIME: 55 MINUTES
SERVES 4–6

500 g carrots, peeled if
   necessary, roughly chopped
3 tablespoons extra virgin
   olive oil, plus extra
   for drizzling
1 brown onion, chopped
2 garlic cloves, chopped
20 g ginger, chopped
1 lemongrass stalk, white part
   only, finely chopped
1 bird's eye chilli, seeded and
   thinly sliced
1 tablespoon Thai curry paste
   (look for one without MSG
   or other additives)
1 teaspoon coriander seeds
2 cups coconut milk
3¼ cups vegetable stock
   (ideally homemade, but
   if store-bought ensure
   it is MSG free)
sea salt and freshly ground
   black pepper
1 x 400 g tin chickpeas,
   drained and rinsed
chopped coriander, to garnish

Preheat the oven to 200°C.

Place the chopped carrot in a roasting tin and toss with half the olive oil. Roast for 20–25 minutes or until lightly golden and tender.

Meanwhile, heat the remaining olive oil in a large saucepan over low heat. Add the onion, garlic, ginger, lemongrass, chilli, curry paste and coriander seeds, and sauté for 5 minutes or until the onion has softened and the spices have released their flavour.

Stir in the roasted carrot, coconut milk and vegetable stock. Increase the heat to medium and bring to the boil, then reduce the heat to low and simmer, covered, for 15–20 minutes or until the carrot is soft. Remove from the heat and season with salt and pepper. Allow to cool slightly, then purée in a blender or with a hand-held blender. Return to the heat, add the chickpeas and heat through gently for about 2 minutes.

Serve the soup hot, garnished with the chopped coriander and drizzled with olive oil.

TIP: *You can replace the carrots with parsnips, sweet potato or pumpkin.*

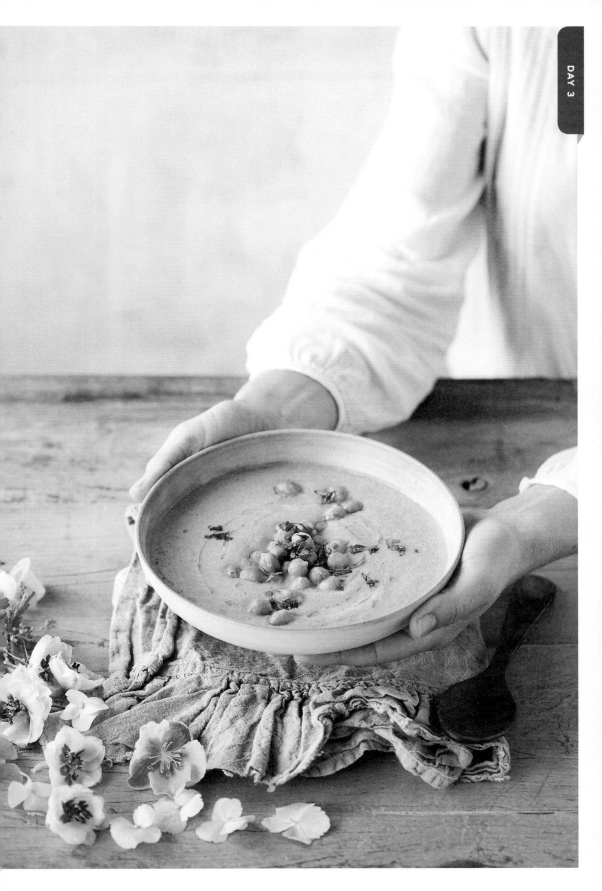

DAY 4

Love your **liver**

If your liver works well, you're lucky. The liver is the body's powerhouse and is responsible for clearing used hormones, balancing blood sugar levels and converting fat into energy – a key to weight loss. It's the body's filter and helps remove fat-soluble toxins, including excess oestrogen. Bile, produced by the liver, helps break down fat, and regulates glucose, blood pressure, insulin, oestrogen, testosterone, immunity and blood cholesterol production and removal. A blood test can reveal if your liver is functioning properly.

Other key signs that your liver is under strain include:

* slightly yellow or discoloured eyes
* pain or discomfort in upper right tummy
* abdominal fat and/or a beer belly
* trouble digesting fatty foods
* gallbladder issues
* acid reflux or heartburn
* acne, rosacea or irritated skin
* inability to lose weight.

If the liver becomes overburdened from excessive food and alcohol, it can't do its job. The metabolism slows and excess hormones remain in the body, creating an imbalance.

WHAT IS FATTY LIVER DISEASE?

Non-alcoholic fatty liver disease (NAFLD) is now seen in adults and children of all ages and is becoming the number one reason for liver transplants (overtaking cirrhosis, which is caused by an overconsumption of alcohol).

NAFLD is also associated with metabolic syndrome, obesity and cardiovascular disease. Obesity is now considered to be a contributing factor, caused by a diet high in sugar, unhealthy fats and processed foods.

TODAY'S ACTION

Assist your liver by eating foods that contain sulfur compounds, including onions, garlic, cabbage, broccoli, brussels sprouts and kale. Help the liver process excess oestrogen with glutathione from avocados, walnuts and asparagus. Vitamin C stimulates the body to produce more glutathione. Drinking even small amounts of alcohol can increase oestrogen levels in the blood because alcohol competes for the available glutathione, preventing oestrogen excretion. Drink plenty of water.

THREE EASY WAYS TO CLEANSE YOUR LIVER

1. **Spice things up** Turmeric protects the liver against toxins and can help prevent damage to liver cells. Add turmeric to soups or to hot water to create a spice tea.
2. **Go green** Green tea contains antioxidants including catechins, which help prevent fat accumulation and promote liver function.
3. **Go nuts for walnuts** These contain high levels of the amino acid L-arginine and the sulfur-containing antioxidant glutathione, which help detoxify the liver and oxygenate the blood.

ASIAN-STYLE BROCCOLI WITH TOFU

Tofu is high in protein and ideal for non-meat lovers. Because it absorbs the flavour of the sauce, it's great to mix and match with different spices, marinades and dressings. Buy organic or non-GMO tofu.

PREPARATION TIME: 10 MINUTES ♥ COOKING TIME: 15 MINUTES
SERVES 2

2 garlic cloves
2 cups small broccoli
   florets, quartered
3 tablespoons extra virgin
   olive oil
225 g organic firm tofu,
   cut into cubes
2 carrots, peeled if necessary,
   thinly sliced
2 teaspoons lemon juice
1 tablespoon tamari
2 tablespoons grated ginger
1 tablespoon rice wine vinegar
chilli flakes, to taste

Crush or finely chop the garlic and set aside for at least 5 minutes (see tip).

Fill the bottom of a steamer with water to a depth of 4 cm and bring to the boil. Steam the broccoli for 4–5 minutes to maximise nutrient retention.

Heat half the olive oil in a wok over medium heat, add the tofu and carrot and stir-fry until lightly golden. Add the broccoli and garlic, and cook for a further 5 minutes.

Toss the stir-fried vegetables and tofu with the remaining ingredients and serve.

TIPS: *Letting the garlic sit after chopping it releases a compound known as allicin, which assists with liver detoxification pathways and cardiovascular health, and reduces inflammation.*

If you prefer a milder garlic taste, add the garlic to the steamer for the final 2 minutes of steaming.

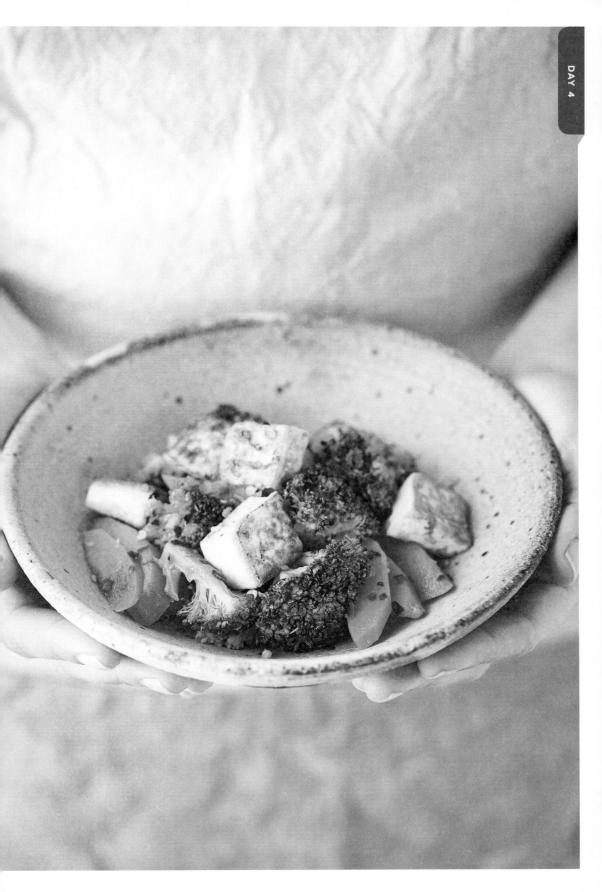

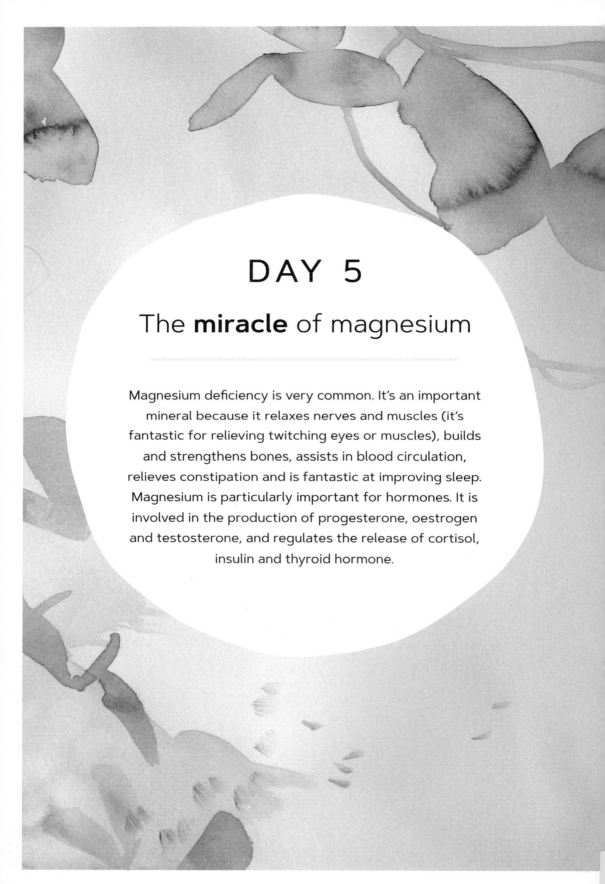

DAY 5

The **miracle** of magnesium

Magnesium deficiency is very common. It's an important mineral because it relaxes nerves and muscles (it's fantastic for relieving twitching eyes or muscles), builds and strengthens bones, assists in blood circulation, relieves constipation and is fantastic at improving sleep. Magnesium is particularly important for hormones. It is involved in the production of progesterone, oestrogen and testosterone, and regulates the release of cortisol, insulin and thyroid hormone.

Magnesium improves mood in women with PMS and helps with insulin sensitivity, metabolic syndrome, prediabetes and diabetes. Because there are several types of magnesium, to work out which is best for you, consult a qualified nutritionist or contact me (see Resources).

Signs of low magnesium include:

* muscle soreness, tremors or spasms. If you exercise, let magnesium be your friend.
* heart arrhythmias, eye twitching or increased heart rate.
* osteoporosis or low bone density. Magnesium and calcium are essential for bone health.
* blood sugar imbalance – it's an excellent nutrient for unstable blood sugar levels.
* headaches – migraines can be relieved by magnesium.
* elevated blood pressure – magnesium is not recommended for those on blood pressure medication because it can cause a drop in blood pressure.
* constipation – magnesium is a gentle way to get your pipes moving without harsh, addictive laxatives.

Many variables affect magnesium in the body. One depleting source is soft drinks. Dark-coloured soft drinks contain phosphates that bind with magnesium in the digestive tract. Rather than being absorbed by the body, the magnesium goes straight through your system unused. When we eat refined sugar, this also makes the body excrete magnesium through the kidneys.

The more sugar you consume, the more likely you are to be deficient in magnesium. Caffeine also leads to more magnesium being released through the kidneys. Age is another factor – magnesium metabolism is less efficient over the age of 55. And stress also affects magnesium levels in the body.

Dark green leafy vegetables are one of the best sources of magnesium. Other good sources include pumpkin seeds, bananas, spinach, dark chocolate (70–85 per cent cocoa), beans, quinoa, oatmeal, brown rice, almonds, cashews, avocado and salmon.

TODAY'S ACTION

Determine the best way to increase the amount of magnesium in your diet and add high-magnesium foods to your plate today. Another way to increase magnesium is by taking a bath in Epsom salts. Soak for 20 minutes and, while you're soaking, drink a cup of magnesium-rich rooibos tea. After bathing, rinse off and prepare for a peaceful night's sleep.

ZUCCHINI SPAGHETTI

Enjoy this 'spaghetti' without the belly bloat. And while it's not the recipe used by my Italian mother, it's delicious all the same. Mushrooms contain energy-giving vitamin B12.

PREPARATION TIME: 15 MINUTES ♥ COOKING TIME: 30 MINUTES
SERVES 4

4 medium zucchini
3 tablespoons extra virgin
    olive oil
4 garlic cloves, crushed
1 cup pine nuts
3 cups roughly
    chopped tomato
2 portobello mushrooms,
    roughly chopped
1 tablespoon dried oregano
1 tablespoon dried thyme
1 cup chopped basil, plus extra
    small leaves to garnish
2 tablespoons honey
2 tablespoons raw
    cacao powder
1 teaspoon sea salt
1 teaspoon freshly ground
    black pepper
nutritional yeast, to serve

Spiralise the zucchini into spaghetti-like noodles, then spread out on paper towel to absorb the excess moisture.

Heat the olive oil in a frying pan over medium heat. Add the garlic and cook for 2 minutes, then add the pine nuts and sauté for 4 minutes. Stir in the tomato, mushroom, oregano, thyme, basil, honey, cacao powder, salt and pepper.

Reduce the heat, then cover and simmer the sauce for 20 minutes, stirring occasionally with a wooden spoon. If you have time, remove the sauce from the heat and let it sit for 2 hours. This will really intensify the flavour.

To serve, divide the spiralised zucchini among four plates, add the sauce and sprinkle with nutritional yeast. Garnish with basil leaves.

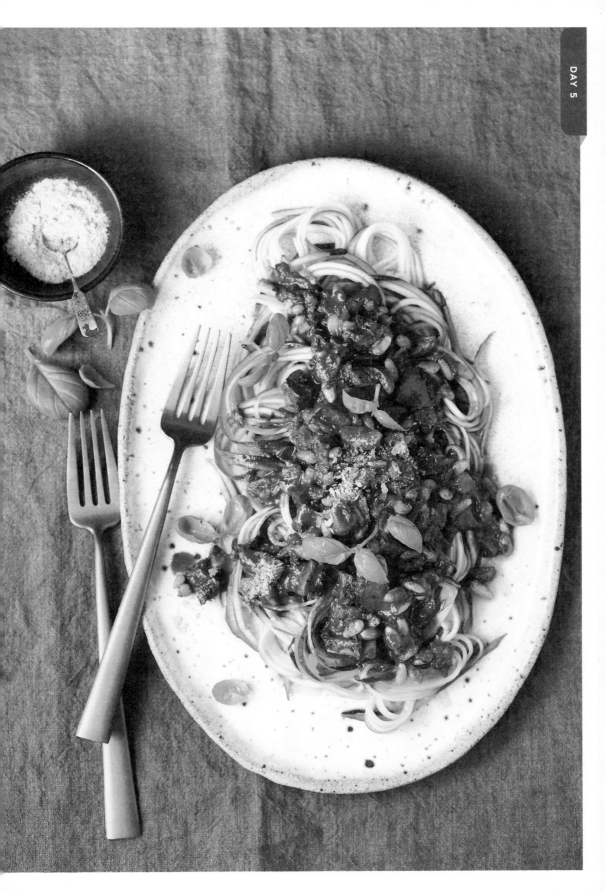

DAY 6

Let's talk about our
new **favourite topic**

If you're struggling and straining on the toilet, you're probably not eating enough fibre. Fibre is the key to regular bowel movements, blood sugar stability, hormone balance and reduced appetite. Fibre helps absorb and eliminate toxins from the colon, including excess oestrogen. It's part of the body's natural detoxification system. When we eat clean, wholesome foods that are rich in fibre, our liver's job is made much easier.

HOW MUCH DIETARY FIBRE SHOULD YOU CONSUME EACH DAY?

The recommended daily intake of fibre is 25–35 grams. If your diet is low in fibre, slowly increase your intake by 5 grams a week until you reach the recommended level. A medium-sized apple has 4.4 grams of fibre, 1 cup of chickpeas has 16 grams of fibre, half an avocado (100 grams) has 6.75 grams of fibre, 1 cup of raspberries has 8 grams of fibre and 100 grams of almonds have 12.5 grams of fibre. Increase fibre by sprinkling whole flaxseeds over your breakfasts and salads. Make sure you thoroughly chew the seeds, or they will pass through your system whole and their nutrients won't be absorbed. The more you chew, the better.

WHAT'S THE BEST TIME OF THE DAY TO HAVE FIBRE?

Eat fibre at any time of the day, with food or on an empty stomach. Ideally, take fibre on its own and wait 30–60 minutes before taking supplements. Drink more water as you increase your fibre intake or you could become constipated. Think about it. If you increase your intake of fibre without increasing your intake of water, you create a gelatinous mass in your intestines that can become stuck. This isn't uncommon. Drink plenty of water and herbal tea, and everything will move smoothly.

In addition to regulating blood pressure, fibre helps LDL or bad cholesterol levels while raising the protective HDL or good cholesterol levels. As a calorie-free weight-loss tool, fibre manages hunger by stimulating the release of cholecystokinin (CCK), a hormone that sends a message to the brain that you're full. High-fibre foods also help normalise blood glucose levels by slowing the time it takes for food to leave the stomach and for glucose to be absorbed from a meal.

Because fibre helps block the absorption of calories and aids in the removal of these calories, think of it as reducing the number of calories in your food. Fibre doesn't break down in the body and isn't converted to sugar, so it doesn't affect blood sugar levels. It reduces cortisol levels and helps to remove excess oestrogen. Those on a high-fibre diet tend to lose weight, improve insulin sensitivity and maintain a healthy body weight. Wonderful, right?

TODAY'S ACTION

My strategy to increase fibre is to add ½–1 teaspoon of whole flaxseeds or chia seeds to yoghurt, salads or smoothies. If you're feeling hard-core, add ½–1 teaspoon of either of these seeds to a large glass of room-temperature water and chew on the seeds as you drink. Do this 30 minutes before a meal, and it will dampen your appetite considerably.

CURRIED CHICKEN ON SPINACH

The vibrant yellow of this dish is from antioxidant-rich turmeric. Turmeric and ginger also contain anti-inflammatory properties that are essential for your overall wellbeing.

PREPARATION TIME: 10 MINUTES ♥ COOKING TIME: 20 MINUTES
SERVES 4

1 tablespoon coconut oil
   or ghee
1 brown onion, halved
   and sliced
3 garlic cloves, sliced
1 teaspoon chopped ginger or
   ½ teaspoon ground ginger
½ teaspoon ground turmeric
1 teaspoon curry powder
3 x 150 g skinless chicken
   breast fillets, cut into
   bite-sized pieces
1 cup chicken stock
   (ideally homemade, but
   if store-bought ensure it
   is MSG free)
1 red capsicum, seeded
   and cut into thin strips
   about 2 cm long
½ cup coconut milk
sea salt and freshly ground
   white pepper
2 large handfuls of
   baby spinach
coriander sprigs, to garnish

Bring a saucepan of water to the boil for the spinach.

Meanwhile, heat the oil or ghee in a frying pan over low–medium heat, add the onion and sauté for about 5 minutes, stirring frequently. Add the garlic and fresh ginger (if using) and sauté for another minute. Add the ground ginger (if using), turmeric and curry powder and mix well. Add the chicken, stock, capsicum and coconut milk and simmer for 10 minutes or until the chicken is cooked through. Season to taste with salt and pepper.

While the chicken is cooking, remove the ends from the spinach and rinse the leaves well, then immerse in the boiling water for 1 minute only. Drain and pat dry with paper towel.

Divide the spinach among four plates and top with the chicken mixture. Garnish with coriander.

TIP: *This recipe can be easily adapted to include more vegetables.*

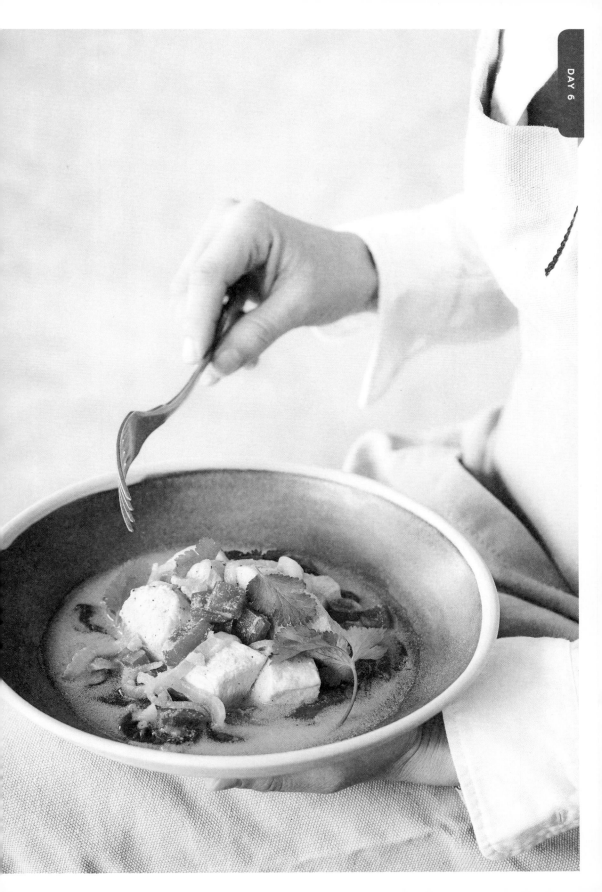

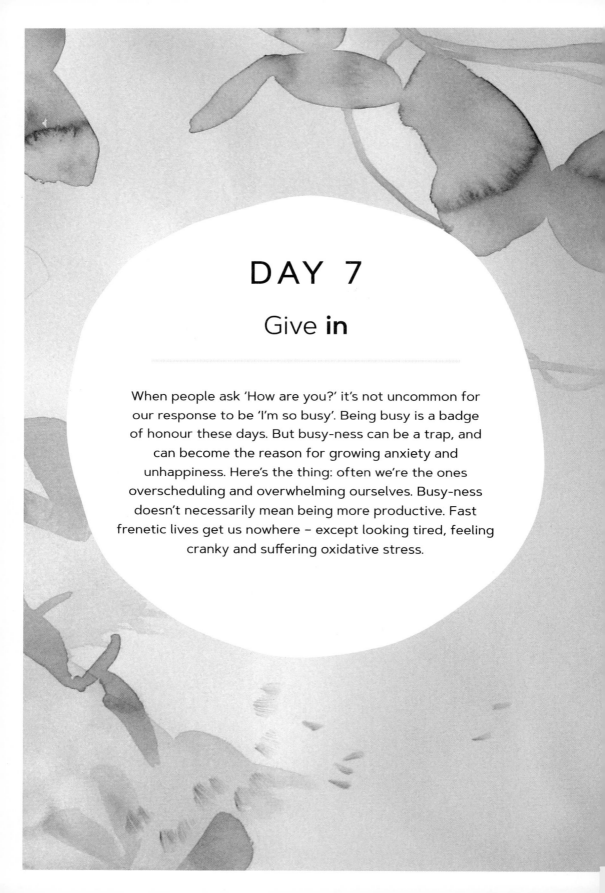

DAY 7

Give **in**

When people ask 'How are you?' it's not uncommon for our response to be 'I'm so busy'. Being busy is a badge of honour these days. But busy-ness can be a trap, and can become the reason for growing anxiety and unhappiness. Here's the thing: often we're the ones overscheduling and overwhelming ourselves. Busy-ness doesn't necessarily mean being more productive. Fast frenetic lives get us nowhere – except looking tired, feeling cranky and suffering oxidative stress.

When we're busy, we're not in the moment. This is the message of Eckhart Tolle's book *The Power of Now.* He writes, 'The only thing that is ultimately real about your journey is the step you are taking at this moment. That's all there ever is.' The past has already happened, the future is still speculation. The only reality is now. One way to come into the present is through your senses – touch, taste, sight, sound and smell. Notice the world through each sense right now. How do you feel?

What happens to your priorities when you're busy? They often fall by the wayside. And one of the first priorities to go is your health. Your plan to go for a walk after work is kicked to the kerb or you skip that early morning exercise class.

Be busy and present, but then find time to give in. Find one hour on both days of this weekend and the following week to simply give in. I know this sounds easy, but it can be more difficult than changing your food habits. It certainly used to be for me. Giving in and nourishing yourself doesn't mean wasting time. Find your own give-in and allow your mind to turn off its chatter and stop pumping out cortisol. The feeling of balance and calm is incredibly beneficial for anti-ageing. Have a bath, go for a swim or a walk, lie in the shade or on the beach, watch a movie or read something uplifting. What's your give-in?

TODAY'S ACTION

This task could be more difficult to achieve than it sounds. Commit to a daily give-in strategy. Take a walk before work. Sit in the sun during lunch. Book yourself in for a massage. I myself enjoy a weekly Thai massage. It's not too expensive – less than the cost of a meal – and there's no need to make a booking. It's easy and works for me. Or you could write in a journal, read or listen to a podcast. Think of this as an anti-ageing strategy.

It took me years to figure out that living life at a mediocre pace doesn't mean living a mediocre life. I now have room for clearer thoughts, better relationships and an abundant heart.

CREAMY CHICKEN CAULIFLOWER CURRY

The protein in this comforting curry satisfies the appetite and the spicy sauce will make your tastebuds dance. Cauliflower is one of the best all-natural detoxifiers.

PREPARATION TIME: 15 MINUTES, PLUS MARINATING TIME
COOKING TIME: 30 MINUTES ♥ SERVES 4

4 x 150 g skinless chicken
   breast fillets
2 teaspoons virgin coconut oil
4 spring onions, white part
   only, finely chopped
1 head cauliflower,
   finely chopped
2½ tablespoons coconut cream
   (optional)
pinch of sea salt
lemon juice, to taste
steamed brown rice, to serve
   (optional)
coriander leaves, to garnish

SAUCE

4 cm piece of ginger, peeled,
   roughly chopped
4 cm piece of turmeric, peeled,
   roughly chopped
2 teaspoons ground cumin
½ teaspoon cayenne pepper
2 pieces preserved lemon rind,
   finely chopped, or finely
   grated zest of 1 lemon
1½ cups coconut cream
pinch of sea salt

To make the sauce, put all the ingredients in a blender and purée until smooth.

Place the chicken breasts in a glass or ceramic dish and pour half the sauce evenly over the top. Leave to marinate for at least 15 minutes.

Preheat the oven to 180°C.

Tear off four large squares of foil and line with similar-sized squares of baking paper. Place one marinated chicken breast on each square, then fold over all sides of the foil to seal it in a parcel. Place the parcels on a baking tray and bake for 25–30 minutes or until the chicken is cooked through. Remove from the oven and set aside.

Meanwhile, heat the coconut oil in a large frying pan over medium heat. Add the spring onion and cauliflower and cook for 2–3 minutes, then stir in the remaining sauce. Simmer for 15 minutes or until the cauliflower is cooked but still firm, adding the coconut cream or a splash of water if the sauce is too thick. Season to taste with salt and lemon juice.

Spoon the cauliflower and rice (if using) onto four plates and add a chicken breast to each. Garnish with coriander and serve.

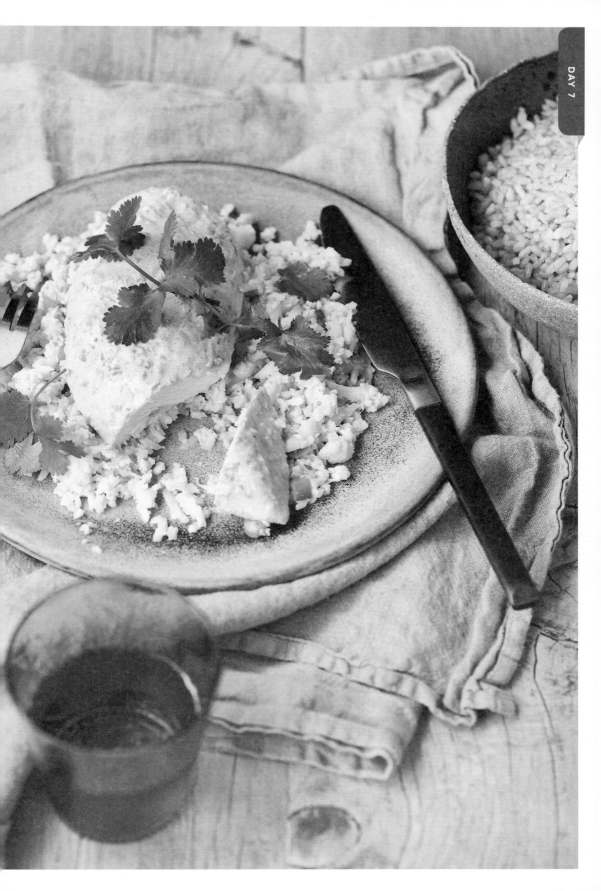

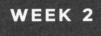

DAY 8

Preparation: the key to creating change

Planning is the key to creating change. If you prepare, I promise you will succeed. Prepare on weekends and at the end of each day. No excuses. Just do it and before you know it, it will become a habit. Positive change is the reason you embarked on this plan, so take today to review and design your next few days. What's on your shopping list? Use the list on page 80 for pointers.

How much time do you need for cooking? Can you cook up a big batch of healthy food, and freeze it in meal-sized portions ready to thaw as needed? Have you made vegetables the centrepiece of your meals? Review the recipes coming up in the next week, create your own or look online for meals that match the five food-combining rules (see page 88). Snap them on your smartphone and create a folder of these favourite go-to meals that satisfy your tastebuds and your hormones.

I often double the quantities of a recipe so I can cook once and eat twice. It doesn't take much extra time to prepare two chicken dishes rather than one. Remember to buy extra storage containers, preferably glass, to use when reheating. Glass is preferable because some plastics contain endocrine disruptors, such as BPA, that can mess with hormones.

When I explain to clients why they need to change their diet and lifestyle, they feel excited. Although they often feel a little daunted at first, once they have a clear reason why they need to change, it helps them to commit. I tell them about other clients who battled low energy, stubborn weight gain and mood swings until they made these changes – and that planning was the cornerstone of their success. Think about it. When was the last time you enjoyed success? Did it take time and planning? The answer is usually yes. Why not apply the same principles to your health? You can have all the money in the world, but if you don't have your health, you don't have quality of life.

Planning means you won't grab the nearest food when the hunger pangs hit. For one thing, you won't have hunger pangs because you're eating three quality meals and two snacks every day. And when temptation comes along, which it will, you won't be caught off guard. Thanks to your excellent planning, you have a range of healthy frozen meals to choose from.

Planning also includes your mindset. What's your strategy if you're out with friends and there's only pizza on the menu? Or at work when birthday cake is offered? Your mindset involves the story you tell yourself about the rebalance. Are you making choices for your health? Or are you telling yourself you're missing out? The rebalance is not about deprivation; it's about eating an abundance of healthy, hormone-stabilising and satiating food.

TODAY'S ACTION

Today there is only one thing you need to do: prepare nourishing meals – nothing more. Oh, and smile. After all, you've been cleansing for seven days.

CLEANSING THAI SOUP

This soup is my all-time 'cleansing high'. Chillies are a 'thermogenic' food
that help to boost your metabolic rate without exercise. How good is that?

PREPARATION TIME: 10 MINUTES ♥ COOKING TIME: 20 MINUTES
SERVES 4

4 x 150 g skinless chicken
  breast fillets
3 cups vegetable stock
  (ideally homemade, but
  if store-bought ensure it
  is MSG free)
3 cups water
2 tablespoons grated ginger
2 garlic cloves, crushed
2 tablespoons tamari
2 bird's eye chillies, seeded
  and finely chopped
2 bunches bok choy
1 red capsicum, seeded
  and thinly sliced
4 spring onions, white part
  only, thinly sliced
½ cup coriander leaves

Combine the chicken, stock, water, ginger, garlic, tamari
and chilli in a large saucepan. Cover and bring to the
boil over high heat, then reduce the heat and simmer,
covered, for 10–15 minutes or until the chicken is
cooked through. Remove the chicken from the stock.
Cover and keep warm.

Return the stock to the heat, stir in the bok choy
and capsicum and simmer until the vegetables are
just tender.

Thickly slice the chicken across the grain. Divide the
broth and vegetables among serving bowls and top with
the chicken. Garnish with the spring onion and coriander
and serve.

TIP: *You can replace the chicken with the same quantity*
      of white fish fillets, such as dory, snapper or cod, skin
      and bones removed. Reduce the cooking time until
      the fish is just cooked through, and flake the fish into
      bite-sized pieces before adding to the broth.

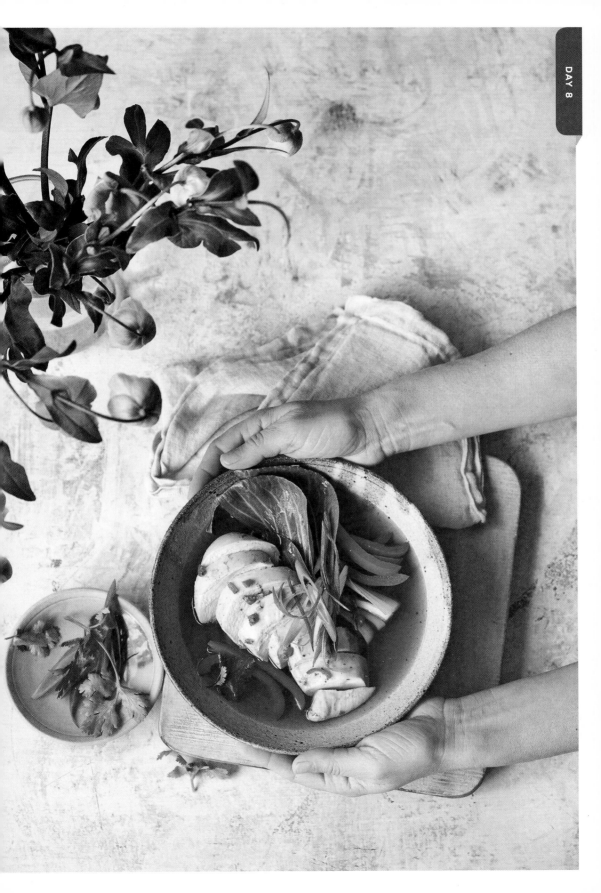

DAY 9

The link between stress, weight and hormones

I know I've already talked about stress, but if you don't have it under control, you won't be able to shift excess weight. Here's a quick reminder of the process: when the body prepares to deal with stress, it releases the hormones adrenaline and cortisol. Both seek out the body's stores of fats and carbohydrates for quick energy. If our body perceives an event as stressful, adrenaline is released, increasing our heart rate, blood pressure, cardiac output and carbohydrate metabolism. Cortisol directs the energy to power our muscles and brain to respond to the stress – whether it's physical or mental.

When the stressful event passes, our adrenaline levels drop off quite quickly, but cortisol sticks around to refuel our body and bring it back into balance. One of the flow-on effects of leftover cortisol is to stimulate our appetite. It wants our body to consume food and replace the fat and carbs used during the real or perceived crisis ('stress-eating').

If stress is sudden and short-lived, our body rebalances. But if we're chronically stressed, our cortisol levels go up and stay up. Chronically elevated cortisol levels can cause other problems, such as depressed immune function, low thyroid function, problems with blood sugar control, adrenal burnout and chronic illnesses such as type 2 diabetes, chronic fatigue and high blood pressure. To drop extra kilos and keep them off, as well as prevent chronic illness, you should do your best to keep your stress levels low (for more on stress, see page 30).

Certain nutrients naturally help us combat stress. These include:

* **zinc** – A deficiency of zinc leads to irritability or chronic anger, poor memory and impaired intellectual ability, loss of taste and smell, and reduced ability to handle stress. Zinc is found in oysters, red meats and poultry, beans, nuts and whole grains.
* **copper** – Copper deficiency causes weakness, digestive issues and breathing problems. Excellent sources of copper are oysters, clams, crab, cashews, hazelnuts, almonds, peanut butter, lentils, beans and whole grains.
* **vitamin B6** – Deficiency can cause irritability, depression, confusion, mouth sores, weakened immune function and intellectual decline. Dietary sources include bananas, salmon, turkey, chicken, potatoes and spinach. To avoid imbalances, B vitamins shouldn't be taken as a single supplement.
* **essential fatty acids (EFAs)** – Deficiencies are linked to decreased memory and mental abilities, nerve tingling, poor vision, lowered immune function, increased LDL or bad cholesterol levels, high blood pressure and irregular heartbeat. They are found in flaxseeds, olive oil, nut oils, walnuts, brazil nuts, avocados, dark leafy greens, salmon, tuna and sesame seeds.

TODAY'S ACTION

Make a list of the ways you can reduce stress in your day. Can you take a 20-minute walk at lunchtime? Can you set your alarm on the hour and breathe deeply for 1 minute? Rather than crashing on the couch after dinner, can you take a walk around the block? There are courses, apps and podcasts on meditation and mindfulness – practices that many high-performance people swear by. Your aim is to prevent cortisol from constantly spiking. To keep your serotonin levels up, eat foods high in tryptophan, such as nuts, seeds, tofu, chicken, turkey, fish, gluten-free oats, cannellini beans, lentils and eggs.

GRILLED OCEAN TROUT WITH DILL BUTTER SAUCE

Don't freak out at the mention of butter sauce. When eaten in moderation, real butter doesn't make you gain weight. The dill butter sauce makes this dish moreish.

PREPARATION TIME: 10 MINUTES ♥ COOKING TIME: 25 MINUTES
SERVES 2

2 pumpkin wedges,
    about 5 mm thick
2 tablespoons extra
    virgin olive oil
2 x 150 g ocean trout or
    salmon fillets, skin and
    bones removed
2 cups salad vegetables
    (such as red onion, tomato,
    olives and cucumber)
2 cups rocket or mixed
    salad leaves

DILL BUTTER SAUCE
60 g butter
juice of ½ lemon
3 tablespoons chopped dill,
    plus extra sprigs, to serve

Preheat the oven to 180°C and line a baking tray with baking paper.

Brush both sides of the pumpkin wedges with half the olive oil and place on the prepared tray. Bake, turning once, for 25 minutes or until tender and golden around the edges.

Meanwhile, preheat an overhead grill to high. Brush both sides of the fish fillets with the remaining olive oil and grill for 3–4 minutes each side. The fish is cooked when the flesh is just starting to fall apart.

To make the dill butter sauce, melt the butter in a small saucepan. Remove from the heat and stir in the lemon juice, then add the dill.

Toss the salad vegetables with the rocket or salad leaves. Divide between two plates and serve with the fish, pumpkin and sauce. Sprinkle with dill sprigs.

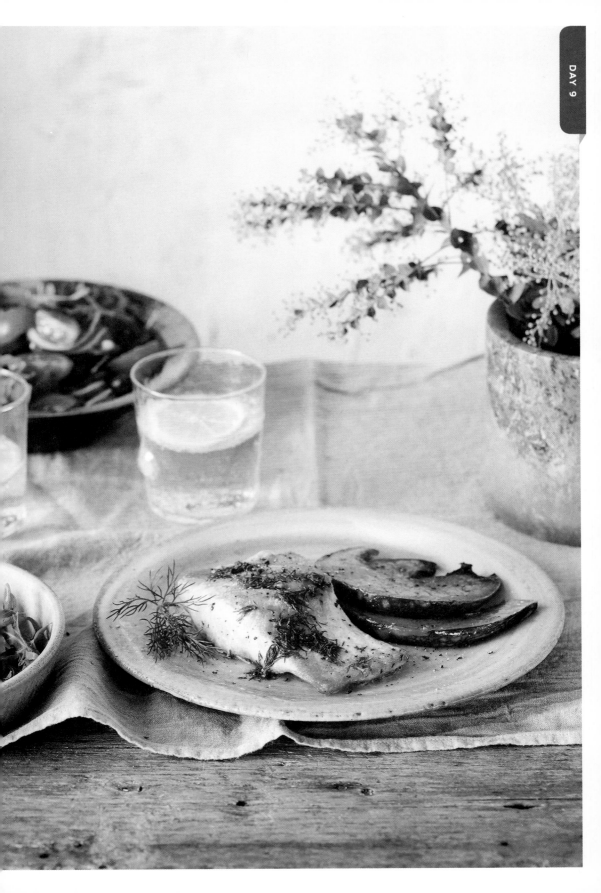

DAY 10

Full-fat or skim?

You should enjoy eating full-fat foods but simply eat less of them. Full-fat foods undergo less processing and make you feel more satiated. Skim milk products are lower in calories and fat but far less tasty. US nutritionist Walter Willett of the Harvard School of Public Health has said, 'The idea that all fats are bad still persists in the minds of many people, despite layers of evidence that this is not true. If anything, low fat/high carbohydrate diets seem to be related to greater long-term weight gain.'

In other words, eating fats isn't specifically related to greater amounts of fat in our bodies. Willett's own research suggests that overall dairy consumption is not substantially related to weight gain or loss, but there is less weight gain from eating full-fat yoghurt. For decades, fat was the subject of a smear campaign, and food manufacturers jumped on board offering low-fat and reduced-fat products. But in order to retain flavour, they often replaced the fat with sugars and salt. You know I don't like most processed foods, but if you do buy them, don't be seduced by the low-fat offerings. Check the label to see if sugars and salt are sky-high.

While carbohydrates are easily digested by the body, fat is not. This means that when we eat fat, we feel fuller for longer. Many people have difficulty accepting this principle. But after one week of eating more fat, most people say they feel full for longer and don't snack as often.

Good-quality fats:

* reduce hunger
* dampen sugar cravings
* improve brain function (our brains are 60 per cent fat)
* assist with hormone balance
* lubricate joints
* are necessary for absorption of the fat-soluble vitamins A, D, E and K.

TODAY'S ACTION

Don't be afraid to eat good fats, but don't go overboard either. As you know, I don't like to count grams or calories, but if you like to work from figures, 30 per cent of your daily calories – or 40–85 grams a day depending on your age, gender and level of activity – can come from good fats. One handful of almonds contains around 30 grams of fat, 1 avocado has 40 grams of fat and 1 tablespoon of oil has 20 grams of fat. Add a quarter of an avocado to your meals, use coconut oil and coconut milk in curries, use good-quality extra virgin olive oils and be generous with your marinades and dressings. Generous enough that your tastebuds are delighted. And generous enough that you don't feel as though you are detoxing, but instead cleansing and rebalancing.

CHILLI CHICKEN STIR-FRY

It's a good idea to double the quantities in this recipe to enjoy as leftovers the next day.
This dish is full of fibre-rich veggies and phytonutrients that are great for skin elasticity.

PREPARATION TIME: 10 MINUTES ♥ COOKING TIME: 15 MINUTES
SERVES 4

1 tablespoon coconut oil
1 brown onion, finely chopped
1 garlic clove, crushed
1 red chilli, seeded and thinly
   sliced, plus extra sliced chilli
   to serve (optional)
4 x 150 g skinless chicken
   breast fillets (or use thigh
   if preferred), sliced
300 g coleslaw mix,
   or shredded cabbage
   and grated carrot
50 g shiitake mushrooms,
   sliced
1 zucchini, finely diced
1 tablespoon tamari
1 tablespoon lime juice
¼ teaspoon sea salt
¼ teaspoon freshly ground
   black pepper
coriander or Thai basil,
   to garnish

Melt the coconut oil in a large wok over high heat. Add the onion, garlic and chilli and stir-fry for 3–4 minutes or until softened.

Add the chicken and stir-fry for 6–7 minutes or until almost cooked through. Add the coleslaw mix, mushrooms and zucchini and stir-fry for 2–3 minutes.

To finish, add the tamari, lime juice, salt and pepper. Garnish with plenty of coriander or Thai basil and serve immediately.

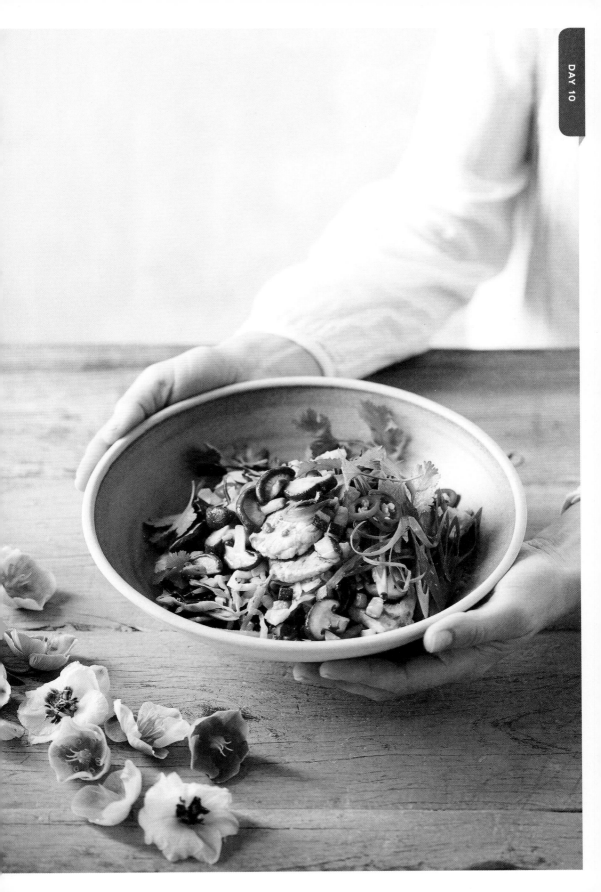

DAY 11

The **importance of sleep**

Good sleep is vital for balanced hormones. As we sleep, protein synthesis takes place, enabling cell repair and growth. Our body recovers from damage caused by stress, cortisol release and ultraviolet rays, and sleep also boosts immunity. Sleep protects our brain, and fights cancer, diabetes, Alzheimer's disease, heart disease and more. When we sleep, we release melatonin, which has a calming effect on our reproductive hormones and protects us against ovarian, endometrial, breast and prostate cancer. Lack of sleep can lower our leptin levels, which makes us hungry.

Several studies suggest that lack of sleep can play a significant role in insulin resistance and type 2 diabetes. In one study, sleep-deprived women were 34 per cent more likely to develop symptoms of diabetes than women who slept seven to eight hours a night. Lack of sleep leads to persistently high cortisol (see page 28 for the effects of this on the body).

TODAY'S ACTION

Consider whether there any impediments to you getting a good night's sleep and work out what you can do to fix them. Create a peaceful bedroom and only use it for sleep – not for work, stress or eating. Go to bed at the same time each night. Eight hours of sleep is ideal, but everyone is different and some people need more and others less.

SEVEN WAYS TO ENHANCE SLEEP

1. **Reduce inflammation** – Chronic inflammation elevates cortisol and agitates the nervous system, which can lead to disturbed sleep. Fish oil and turmeric can reduce inflammation in the body.
2. **Embrace magnesium** – Magnesium calms the body. It's found in whole foods such as green leafy vegetables, seeds and nuts.
3. **Go for glutamine** – The body converts glutamine to gamma-aminobutyric acid (GABA), a calming sleep-promoting neurotransmitter. Sources include unsweetened yoghurt, chicken, beef and fish.
4. **Don't starve** – This rebalance is designed to prevent hunger. An agitated, hungry person doesn't sleep well.
5. **Avoid stimulants and depressants** – Alcohol and caffeine can interfere with the quality of sleep. Drinking alcohol makes you feel tired but it interrupts REM sleep and can wake you up in the middle of the night. Caffeine is a stimulant and diuretic.
6. **Reduce liquids** – After 6 pm, limit the amount of water, juice, tea and other fluids you drink to minimise the need for toilet trips throughout the night.
7. **Drink alkalising minerals** – These minerals, such as potassium citrate, calm the nervous system. Sources include strawberries and avocados. Coconut water is also high in potassium, but because it's very sweet and I want you to dampen your sweet tastebuds, don't drink it during the rebalance.

CHICKEN VEGETABLE SOUP

Chicken soup is good for the soul and the waistline. Celery is a wonderful diuretic with an abundance of fibre.

PREPARATION TIME: 20 MINUTES ♥ COOKING TIME: 1 HOUR 20 MINUTES
SERVES 4–6

1 x 1.2–1.8 kg chicken
2 tablespoons extra virgin
   olive oil
1 leek, white part only,
   halved lengthways,
   washed and thinly sliced
2 garlic cloves, crushed
1 large carrot, peeled if
   necessary, diced
4 celery stalks, diced
2 small zucchini, diced
1 turnip, peeled and diced
2 litres chicken stock
   (ideally homemade, but
   if store-bought ensure it
   is MSG free)
2 cups cold water
sea salt and freshly ground
   black pepper
chilli flakes and chopped
   flat-leaf parsley, to serve

Wash the chicken and pat dry with paper towel.

Heat the olive oil in a saucepan large enough to hold the chicken over medium heat. Add the leek and garlic and sauté for 2 minutes or until soft but not coloured. Add the carrot, celery, zucchini and turnip and sauté for 2 minutes.

Add the chicken, stock and cold water, ensuring the chicken is covered with liquid (add more water if needed). Increase the heat to high and bring to the boil, then reduce the heat to low and simmer, partially covered, for 1 hour or until the vegetables are tender and the chicken is cooked through and nearly falling off the bone, stirring occasionally.

Carefully remove the chicken from the soup and allow to cool slightly. Skim away any skin or froth that may have settled on the surface of the soup. Remove the meat from the bones and roughly chop, then return it to the soup. Season with salt and pepper.

Ladle the soup into warmed bowls, scatter over the chilli flakes and parsley, and serve.

TIP: *You can reduce the cooking time if you use a pre-cooked free-range barbecued chicken. Gently pull the meat off the bones and add to the soup after it has been simmering for about 20–30 minutes. Serve warm.*

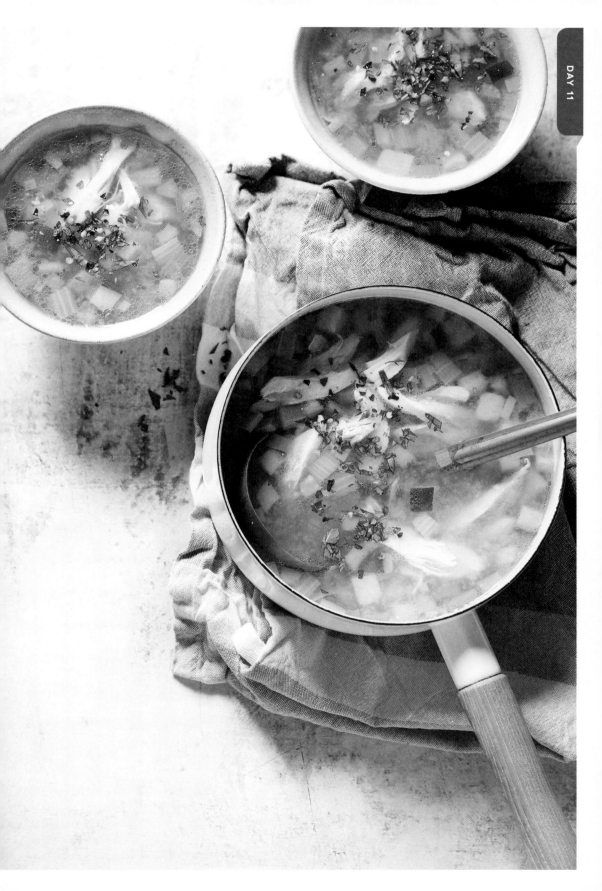

DAY 12

How **thirst affects cortisol**

You might think you're hungry when you're really just thirsty. When we're dehydrated, our body registers this as stress. It releases cortisol, which releases glucose, and because it's in excess it's eventually stored as fat. Lack of hydration can also make you feel lethargic, which makes sense given that 60 per cent of the body is water. Start your day – before your morning toilet stop – with a glass of not-too-cold water with a squeeze of lemon or lime.

One way to work out if you're drinking enough is to check the colour of your urine. The paler the yellow, the better. Darker yellow is a sign you need to drink more water. If you've been exercising, you need to up the hydration or you could suffer from muscle fatigue. One suggestion is to drink a glass of water at the same time and same place each day – that way, it will soon become a habit you won't have to think about. Buy a water bottle you love and swig from it during the day. Some people turn drinking water into a game and compete with family or colleagues by recording their drinking units to see who drinks the most.

Among its many benefits, water:

* helps speed up metabolism and assists with weight reduction
* can improve energy by keeping the blood transporting oxygen and other nutrients to cells
* keeps your digestion moving, especially in conjunction with fibre. If you don't drink enough water, the colon takes water from poo, which can cause constipation.

Rehydrate with herbal teas such as licorice tea or cinnamon tea, or still or sparkling water. I also recommend drinking one or two cups of green tea per day. Even though it contains caffeine, the amounts are negligible. If you don't like the taste, disguise it by combining it with flavours you love.

TODAY'S ACTION

Today, focus on hydration. Choose a favourite teacup or water bottle. (It may sound silly, but when you have a teacup or water bottle you love, it makes drinking much more pleasant and enjoyable.) Have a range of herbal teas to choose from. Keep a glass jug filled with water on your kitchen bench or desk at work, and add slices of lemon or lime, berries and/or mint leaves to make it inviting. If you often visit the toilet in the middle of the night and find it difficult to get back to sleep, I suggest limiting the amount you drink from 4 pm. You want to enjoy the restorative effect of a full night's sleep.

In a couple of weeks, you'll look in the mirror and think: 'I have fewer fine lines, no dark circles under my eyes and my skin is glowing.' Hydration is vital, and happens from the inside out. Dehydration makes your skin look more wrinkled.

VEGETABLE FRITTATA

*In my opinion, eggs are the best source of protein. They are full of amino acids,
which are the building blocks for lean muscle mass. Flavourful leeks are a great
prebiotic food. I love a dish that gives so much.*

PREPARATION TIME: 15 MINUTES ♥ COOKING TIME: 25 MINUTES
SERVES 4–6

40 g butter
3 leeks, white part only,
   halved lengthways,
   washed and thinly sliced
2 organic eggs
10 organic egg whites
1 teaspoon finely chopped chilli
sea salt and freshly ground
   black pepper
250 g drained frozen spinach
1 cup cherry tomatoes, halved
basil leaves, to serve
1 avocado, cut into 4–6 pieces,
   or Healthy Guacamole (see
   page 217), to serve

Preheat the oven to 180°C.

Melt the butter in a large ovenproof non-stick frying pan over medium heat, add the leek and sauté for about 10 minutes or until it starts to caramelise.

Meanwhile, in a large bowl, whisk the eggs, egg whites and chilli for about 2 minutes. Add a generous pinch each of salt and pepper.

Squeeze as much water as you can from the spinach.

Spread out the leek over the base of the pan and pour over the egg mixture. Scatter over the spinach and leave the mixture to sit for a minute or two, until the egg is just set at the edges. Using a spatula, lift the sides to check the underside is becoming firm enough to hold the tomatoes.

As it starts to firm more, lay the tomatoes on top, cut-side up. Transfer the pan to the top shelf of the oven and cook for about 8 minutes. It should be set but still have a little give when you push it in the middle. If you want to brown the top, put it under a hot grill for a minute or so.

Remove the frittata from the oven and allow to cool slightly, then scatter over the basil and season to taste with salt and pepper. Serve with the avocado or guacamole.

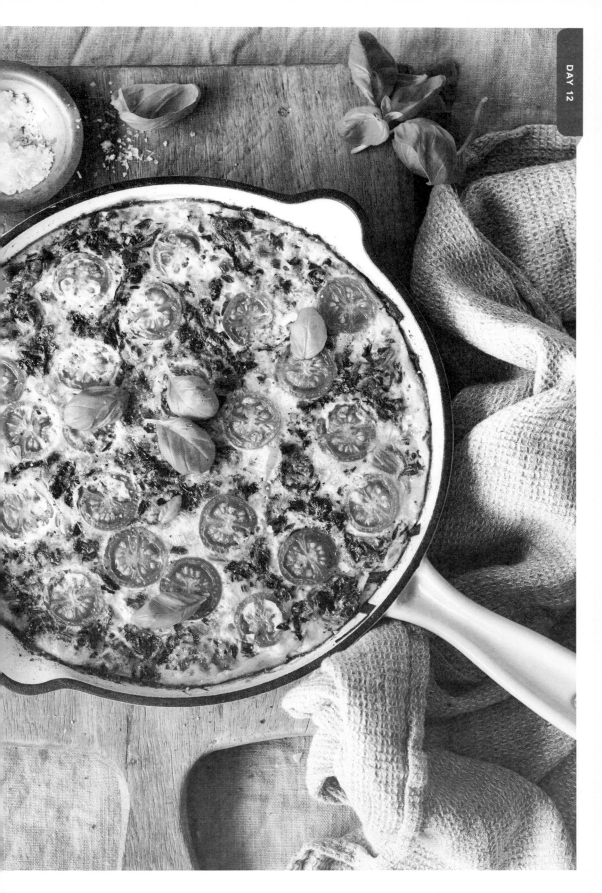

DAY 13

The **happy** hormone, **serotonin**

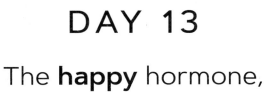

As outlined earlier, serotonin plays an important
role in balanced moods. It's manufactured in both the brain
and the intestines; in fact, 90 per cent of the body's
serotonin is synthesised in the gastrointestinal tract.
The gut is now referred to as the 'second brain', and it
makes sense that tummy issues will affect your mood.
Serotonin is an active area of research and scientists
are not sure if lower levels of serotonin contribute
to depression or if depression causes lower
levels of serotonin.

Serotonin is important because it:

* influences appetite regulation
* helps balance insulin and its opposing hormone, glucagon, for normal blood glucose levels
* assists with sleep
* affects cortisol release.

The cleaner your diet, the more balanced your serotonin levels. People with low serotonin often consume greater amounts of sugar in an attempt to boost serotonin production. If you're feeling low, sugar can make you feel better, but the feeling is only temporary. If your inner critic starts speaking, it can be easy to silence it with sugar. It's easier to eat unhealthy food than it is to deal with difficult emotions. But using sweet and processed food to numb pain is neither healthy nor sustainable, and won't get you any closer to your clean slate.

When you experience overwhelming cravings, it could indicate unbalanced blood sugar levels, mixed signalling from hormones, a lack of nutrients or a learned emotional response. Low blood sugar and low serotonin tell the brain you want a sugar hit. If you use caffeine to power you through the day, it releases cortisol, which releases glucose, which in turn tells the brain you want a sugar hit. Are you seeing a pattern here? The best tool to fight back against cravings is to eat three balanced meals and two snacks a day. If you skip, you dip and you crave. And it all goes pear-shaped. When the rebalance becomes habitual, you can skip morning tea or afternoon tea. But for now, stick to three meals and two snacks a day.

TODAY'S ACTION

If your gut is happy and functional, there'll be an improvement in your serotonin levels. The rebalance removes serotonin-reducing culprits such as sugary, high-carb processed foods; soft drinks; and foods with a high GI, such as white bread and dried fruit. Alcohol also reduces serotonin. A great way to increase serotonin is through exercise, and a good intake of healthy fats is also in order. Smile. Be kind to yourself. Give yourself a pat on the back. It's almost two weeks since you started the rebalance.

I'm a nutritionist who tells people to eat more, not less. If you skip a meal or snack, your blood sugar can dip, especially as you're getting used to this new way of life. Don't skip and you won't dip. A dip often leads to the dangerous desire to grab sugar.

HERBED WILD-CAUGHT SALMON SALAD

*I love simplicity and freshness, but when you don't have time, it's fine
to reach for a protein-rich tin of salmon or tuna. Chopped herbs contain
phytonutrients that feed the skin and enhance the immune system.*

PREPARATION TIME: 15 MINUTES ♥ COOKING TIME: NIL
SERVES 2

1 x 210 g tin wild-caught
   salmon, drained
3 tablespoons lemon or
   lime juice
2 celery stalks, thinly sliced
½ small fennel bulb,
   thinly sliced
2–3 spring onions, thinly sliced
⅓ cup finely chopped herbs
   (such as basil, flat-leaf
   parsley and coriander)
sea salt and freshly ground
   black pepper
1 cup chopped baby spinach
   or rocket
good-quality extra virgin olive
   oil, for drizzling

Break up the salmon in a medium bowl, add the juice,
celery, fennel, spring onion and herbs and season with
salt and pepper. Toss together, then leave to marinate
for 5 minutes.

Divide the spinach or rocket between two plates and
top with the salmon salad. Finish with a drizzle of olive
oil and serve.

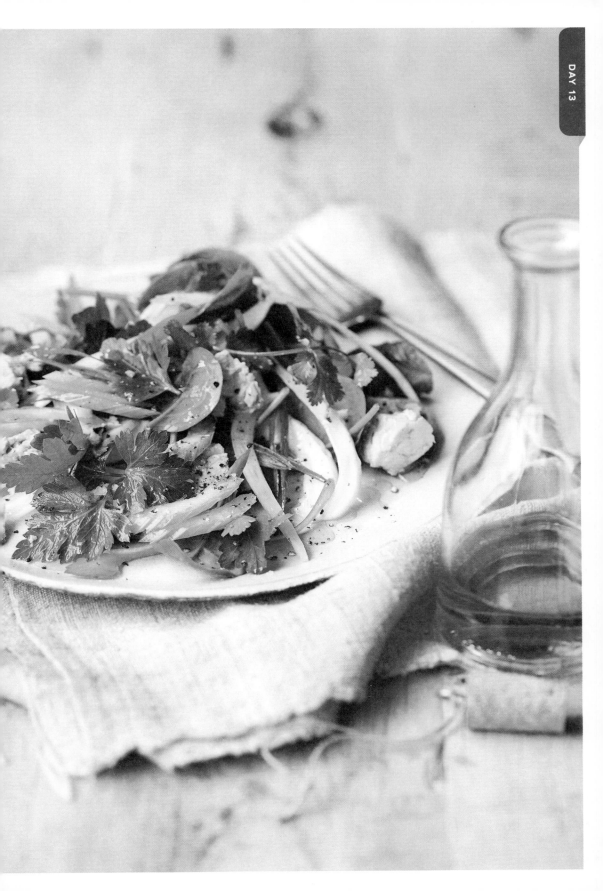

DAY 14

Emotional eating

It's clear that overeating and drinking too much cause weight gain. But there can be other drivers of the 'Betty back fat', 'tummy tube' or 'love muffin' making your clothes feel too tight. One of the most reliable paths to poor eating is stress eating. Stress changes our appetite, stimulates overeating and increases insulin resistance. Women often overeat for emotional reasons rather than hunger. Emotional eating blunts the reward response in the brain, stimulates cortisol and drives cravings.

In his book *The Power of Habit*, **Charles Duhigg describes the realisation he had a 'cookie habit'.** Every day between 3 and 3.30 pm, Charles would rise from his desk at *The New York Times* and head to the office cafeteria to eat a chocolate chip cookie. After gaining 3.6 kilograms, he examined this habit and realised that what he was seeking was not a sugar hit, but a chance to take a break from his work, chat with colleagues and socialise. It was emotional cookie eating. Once Charles realised he could chat with colleagues without eating cookies yet feel just as satisfied, his urge to eat the cookies disappeared.

If your cravings aren't related to food, I encourage you to look deeper and find out what void you're trying to fill. What do you really need? Do you have cravings because you're hungry, tired, thirsty, bored, lonely, overwhelmed or stressed? A binge on junk food is only going to make you feel worse. Look for the root cause of your cravings. Take notes. Do your cravings happen if you've had a bad night's sleep? Or because you feel overwhelmed by a family situation you can't control? Or feel stressed at work? Or feel unloved or unappreciated? Or because you're bored and uninspired by your work or life? Or simply lacking in nutrients? Once you note what's driving your cravings, consider how you can manage them. Do you need more sleep, a resolution of family issues, a new job? Talk about how you feel. Find joy. Eat regularly. Remain hydrated. If you decide to give in to cravings, have a list of foods and drinks you can indulge in, such as licorice tea or cinnamon tea, a bowl of berries, chia seed pudding, iced tea with a pinch of stevia and a squeeze of lemon or lime juice, or a handful of your favourite nuts.

TODAY'S ACTION

Today, become aware what you're thinking before you reach into the fridge or pantry. Are you eating because you're sad, bored, frustrated or hungry? If so, acknowledge that you're stressed or depressed and do something about it. Seek out supportive friends, start a new sport, or practise yoga or meditation. Take up a hobby that keeps your hands busy, like sewing or carpentry, or doing a crossword or Sudoku. Discover what you really need. The vicious circle of overeating then beating yourself up is destructive. And remember, you're the one in control.

TASTY THAI CHICKEN CAKES

Even the fussiest eaters will love this meal disguised as a muffin. Chicken thigh meat is higher in iron than breast meat — a key mineral that underpins physical and mental energy.

PREPARATION TIME: 15 MINUTES ♥ COOKING TIME: 15 MINUTES
SERVES 4

coconut oil, for greasing
500 g skinless chicken thigh
    fillets, roughly chopped
2 garlic cloves,
    roughly chopped
large handful of baby spinach
2 teaspoons wheat-free
    fish sauce or tamari
3 teaspoons coconut cream
1 teaspoon chopped ginger
Healthy Guacamole (see page
    217) or Simple Spicy Slaw
    (see page 166), to serve
coriander sprigs and lime
    wedges, to garnish

Preheat the oven to 180°C and grease eight holes of a muffin tin with coconut oil.

Place the chicken, garlic, spinach, fish sauce or tamari, coconut cream and ginger in a food processor and pulse until well combined but not entirely smooth. A little texture is good.

Spoon the mixture evenly into the prepared muffin holes and bake for 15 minutes or until firm. Cool in the tin for a few minutes, then turn out onto a wire rack.

Serve hot or cold with the guacamole or slaw. Garnish with coriander sprigs and lime wedges.

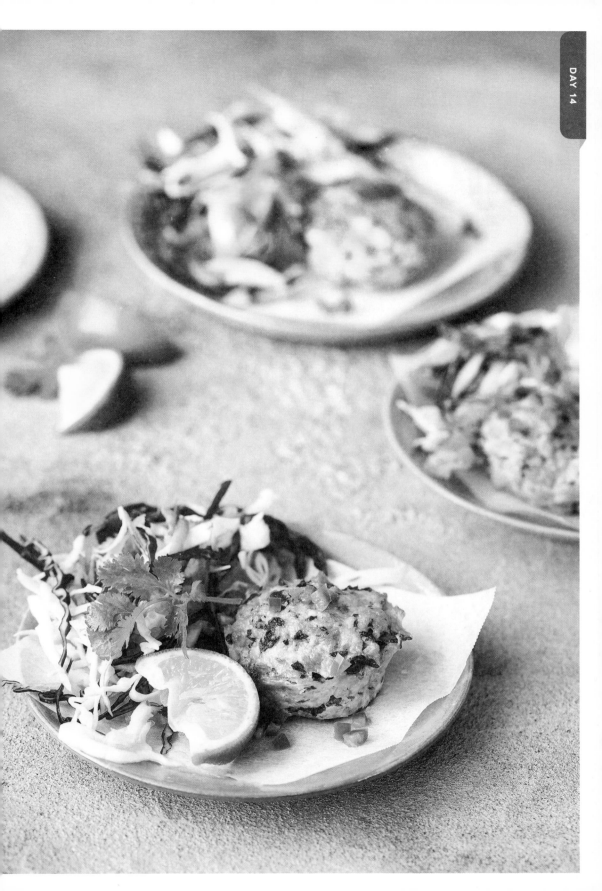

DAY 15

Try **intermittent** fasting

Now that you've established a routine of eating regularly, not feeling hungry and crowding in new foods, I want to shake things up a bit. Starting today, I'd like you to try intermittent fasting by skipping one dinner (no more) each week. Intermittent fasting has been used by nutritionists and endocrinologists for many years, but it has become popular recently thanks to Michael Mosley and his 5:2 diet. When he reduced his calorie intake on two days of each week, it improved his insulin response.

My approach is slightly different: reduce your calorie intake for one meal each week – preferably dinner. I've seen many people do well on the 5:2 diet, but others don't find it sustainable. They lose weight at the beginning but yoyo back to their previous weight. If I was limited to eating only 500 calories a day, I would chew my fingers off and become cranky or 'hangry' – hungry and angry at the same time. Instead of an extreme approach, make your evening meal a bowl of broth or a bowl of non-starchy veggies or skip the meal entirely. Make it an early meal – around 6 pm – to maximise fasting time. You can drink a cup of herbal tea to see you through the evening. The following morning, after 7 am, eat a delicious breakfast. This will wake your insulin receptors.

Fasting has been shown to reduce oxidative stress and inflammation in some people. When cells are under stress, they adapt to that stress. During intermittent fasting, levels of insulin drop, giving the body a break from insulin spikes and crashes. Some people enjoy the feeling they get from an intermittent fast, but it doesn't work for everyone, and research is still in its infancy. It can feel uncomfortable for the first or second time, but then you should feel lightness, energy and clarity. If it really makes you feel stressed or 'hangry', there's no need to skip a meal again. But if you feel better after intermittent fasting, continue to skip one meal each week.

TODAY'S ACTION

Today, if you're feeling good, skip dinner completely or eat only a bowl of broth or non-starchy veggies. Don't fast more than once a week, because there can be a rebound effect of hunger and bingeing. The next morning, write down how you feel. Do you feel light? Bright? Does your tummy feel flatter?

Fasting is a great tool for weight control. There are several ways to practise intermittent fasting, but this approach is modest and non-extreme, and is very effective.

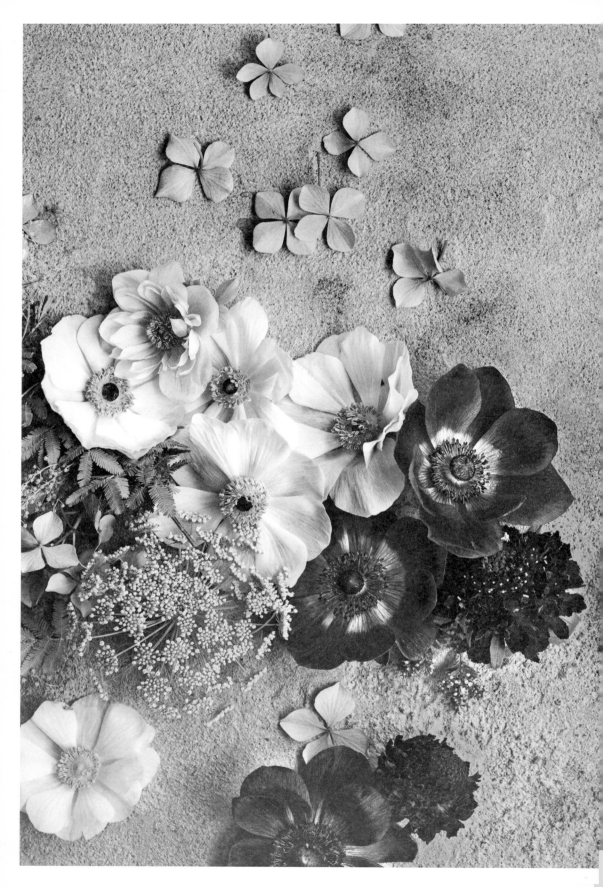

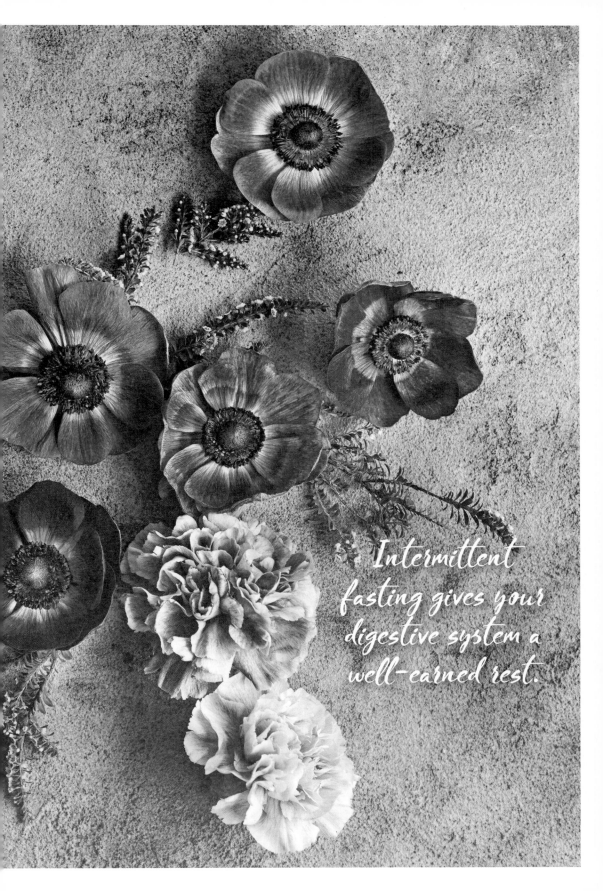

Intermittent
fasting gives your
digestive system a
well-earned rest.

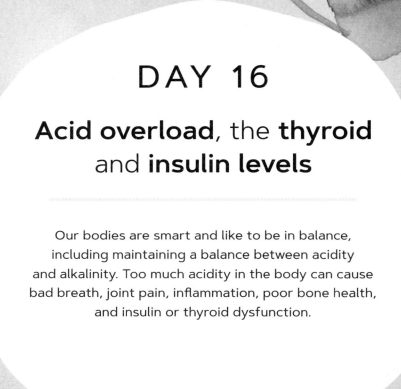

DAY 16

Acid overload, the thyroid and insulin levels

Our bodies are smart and like to be in balance,
including maintaining a balance between acidity
and alkalinity. Too much acidity in the body can cause
bad breath, joint pain, inflammation, poor bone health,
and insulin or thyroid dysfunction.

Processed foods, excessive protein, coffee, alcohol, stress, shallow breathing or poor sleep may push the body into an acidic state. Acidity is also associated with allergies, frequent colds, fatigue, mood swings, irritability and insomnia. Too much acidity can also lead to excess oestrogen.

Acidity is measured using the pH scale, which ranges from 0 to 14, where 7 is neutral, above 7 is alkaline and below 7 is acidic. Our blood pH is 7.35, and to balance excess acidity, the body pulls alkaline minerals such as calcium from storage sites in our bones. This can cause low bone density and osteoporosis. You can test your pH using urine pH strips – a healthy range is between 6.5–7.0.

Carrying extra weight can create acidity in the body, which makes the body produce more insulin. And we know what happens to the body when there are regular insulin spikes and crashes – it puts down belly fat. Processed foods, caffeine and alcohol also contribute to acidity in the body. These foods are off the list already for the rebalance, but other foods on the permitted list can contribute to acidity too. You don't have to cut them out, but you do need to balance them by eating fruit and veggies, which reduce acidity. It's all about creating a balance.

TODAY'S ACTION

Ensure your meals include lots of vegetables, especially green ones. Veggies are the key to health. Fruit and veggies contain essential doses of potassium, calcium and magnesium that keep the body in balance. Most processed foods are acidic, whereas fresh, natural foods are alkaline. The easiest way to ensure pH balance is to eat vegetables when you eat protein foods.

Start the day with a glass of water with a squeeze of lemon juice added. When lemon is metabolised by the body, the effect is alkalising.

MOROCCAN SPICED FISH WITH PEA PURÉE

This dish is fun and tasty. For those who don't love the flavour of fish, it's disguised by antioxidant-rich spices. Edamame and pea mash add additional protein and smart carb energy.

PREPARATION TIME: 15 MINUTES ♥ COOKING TIME: 20 MINUTES
SERVES 4

4 x 150 g white fish fillets
(such as snapper), skin
and bones removed
1 tablespoon Moroccan
spice blend
3 tablespoons extra virgin
olive oil
2 garlic cloves, thinly sliced
4 zucchini, halved lengthways
then sliced
200 g baby spinach
1 teaspoon sea salt
1 teaspoon freshly ground
black pepper
lemon wedges, to serve

PEA PURÉE

1 cup frozen podded edamame
1 cup frozen baby peas
2 tablespoons extra virgin
olive oil

Season the fish fillets with the Moroccan spice blend.

Heat 2 tablespoons of olive oil in a frying pan over medium heat, add the fish and cook for 5 minutes each side. Remove and cover to keep warm.

Heat the remaining olive oil in the same pan and sauté the garlic for 1 minute. Add the zucchini and cook for 5 minutes or until golden, then add the spinach, salt and pepper and sauté for another minute.

Meanwhile, to make the pea purée, bring a medium saucepan of water to the boil. Add the edamame and cook for 1–2 minutes. Add the peas and cook for a further 2–3 minutes or until both the edamame and peas are tender. Drain and place in a blender with the olive oil and blend until smooth.

Spoon the pea purée onto four plates and top with the green vegetable mixture and fish fillets. Serve with lemon wedges.

TIP: *If you don't have any Moroccan spice blend, just replace it with salt and pepper. The fish will still be delicious.*

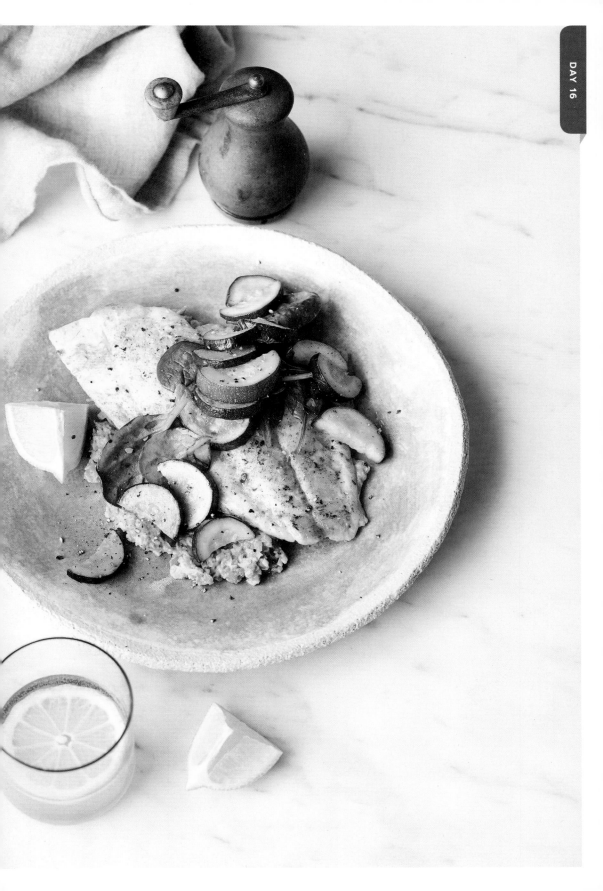

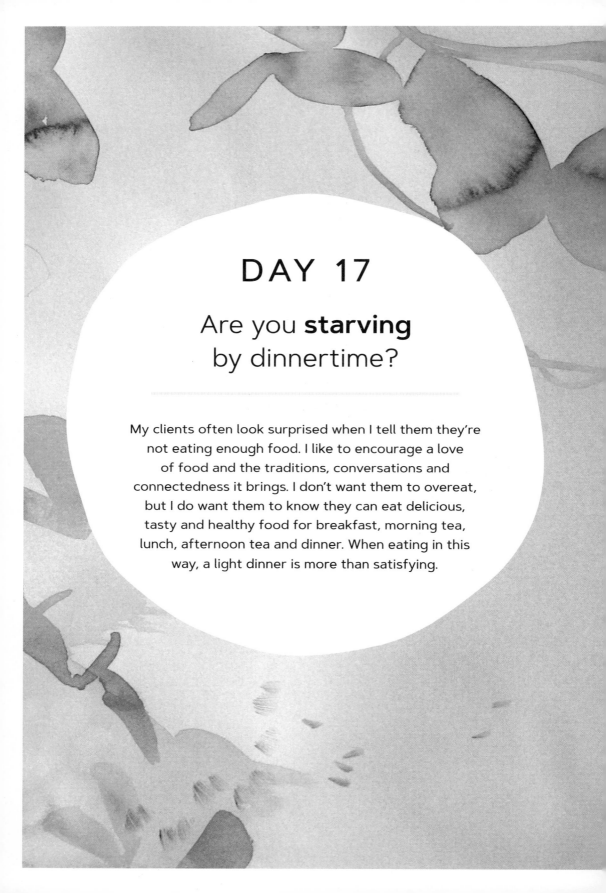

DAY 17

Are you **starving** by dinnertime?

My clients often look surprised when I tell them they're not eating enough food. I like to encourage a love of food and the traditions, conversations and connectedness it brings. I don't want them to overeat, but I do want them to know they can eat delicious, tasty and healthy food for breakfast, morning tea, lunch, afternoon tea and dinner. When eating in this way, a light dinner is more than satisfying.

In my former life, one of my worst habits was eating very little during the day and then eating whatever I could get my hands on during the evening. It meant I wasn't fuelling my brain or body but I was burning out my adrenal glands. When I learned how to shift my weight and lift my energy and mood with food, I realised that eating throughout the day was essential to my vitality, energy levels and brain productivity.

Take note of when you feel hungriest. If you're starving by dinner, you might not be eating enough during the day. This is common with busy people who eat too little throughout the day. When you eat too many calories at dinner and aren't hungry at breakfast, this compounds your problem. The US National Institute on Aging found that middle-aged people who ate their daily calories at dinner produced more ghrelin, the hunger hormone, than when they ate the same calories spread throughout the day. Have a meal or snack every three to four hours. When transitioning to new eating patterns, it's important to eat three meals and two snacks every day even if you don't feel hungry. I don't want you to suddenly feel ravenous. 'Hangry' – hungry and angry – people often grab what's easiest rather than what's healthiest. Trust me on this. Stick with the plan of three meals and two snacks per day and after the rebalance, you can drop the morning and afternoon snacks.

TODAY'S ACTION

Eat bigger meals at breakfast and lunch and a smaller one at dinner. It will take time to become used to the change. You don't want to go to bed on a full stomach. Aim for lightness at dinner and notice how light and energetic you feel the following morning.

SIMPLE SPICY SLAW

I love the taste of spicy slaw and it's so good for you. Cabbage is a natural liver cleanser and fennel offers fibre and slight sweetness. It's excellent for digestion.

PREPARATION TIME: 15 MINUTES ♥ COOKING TIME: NIL
SERVES 4

½ red cabbage, shredded
¼ green cabbage, shredded
1 bunch coriander, finely
   chopped, plus extra
   sprigs to serve
1 carrot, peeled if necessary,
   grated
1 large fennel bulb,
   trimmed and grated
1 jalapeno chilli, seeded
   and finely chopped
1 teaspoon grated ginger
juice of 3 limes
3 teaspoons olive oil
2 teaspoons apple
   cider vinegar
½ teaspoon sea salt

Combine the cabbage, coriander, carrot, fennel, chilli and ginger in a large bowl.

Mix the lime juice, olive oil and vinegar in a small bowl, then toss through the veggies. Sprinkle over the salt and garnish with coriander sprigs.

Serve the slaw with a piece of grilled fish or barbecued chicken.

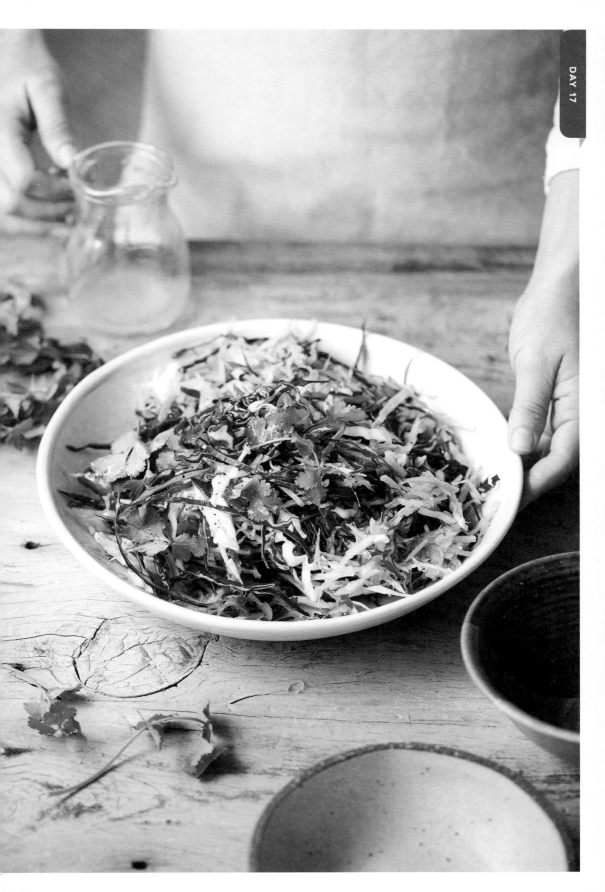

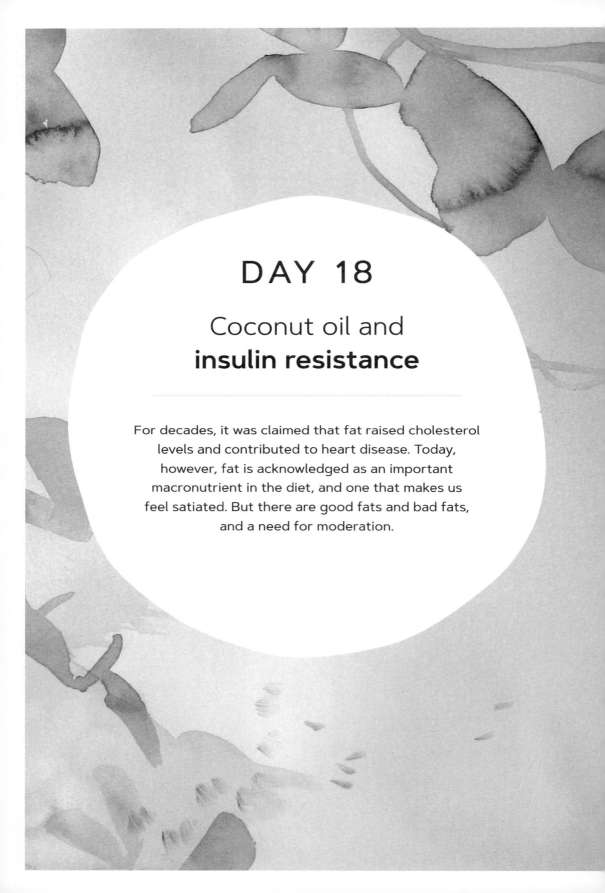

DAY 18

Coconut oil and
insulin resistance

For decades, it was claimed that fat raised cholesterol levels and contributed to heart disease. Today, however, fat is acknowledged as an important macronutrient in the diet, and one that makes us feel satiated. But there are good fats and bad fats, and a need for moderation.

I like cooking with coconut oil. As a largely saturated fat, it doesn't oxidise as easily as other fats, making it ideal to cook with, and it doesn't lose its nutritional value at a high temperature. Because it contains lots of medium-chain fatty acids (MCFAs), it doesn't negatively impact on cholesterol. The body metabolises the MCFAs in the liver and immediately converts them into energy to be used as fuel for the brain and muscles. Coconut oil is also high in lauric acid, which has antiviral and antibacterial properties that can guard against irritable bowel syndrome, Candida and parasites that affect digestion.

Peer-reviewed scholarly research into the health claims of coconut oil is limited and often conducted on rats and mice, but there does seem to be an interesting link between coconut oil and insulin resistance. In one study, rats on a high-fructose diet were fed either copra oil, derived from dried coconut flesh, or virgin coconut oil, derived from fresh coconut flesh and high in antioxidants. Those fed the virgin coconut oil showed improved glucose metabolism. Researchers from Sydney's Garvan Institute of Medical Research compared fat metabolism and insulin resistance in mice that were fed a diet based on either coconut oil or lard. They concluded that the MCFAs in coconut oil can help prevent insulin resistance.

Both ghee and coconut oil are ideal for cooking at high temperatures. Use olive oil for sautéing at moderate temperatures and cold in dressings.

TODAY'S ACTION

If you're craving sweet food in the afternoon, eat a teaspoon of virgin coconut oil, either straight from the spoon or in a cup of green tea. Quality oils are more satiating than carbs. If you're hungry all the time, it means you're not eating well enough. Rather than specify the ratios of fat, protein and carbs during the rebalance, I prefer to look at the ratio of fat, protein and complex carbs from plant sources. In my experience, a ratio of 30 per cent good fats, 30 per cent good-quality protein and 40 per cent smart carbs keeps you satiated, blunts cravings and leads to sustainable weight loss and wellbeing. For oils and fats, that's around 2 tablespoons each meal.

HOLY SWEET POTATO BURGER

Sweet potato is one of the best slow carbs and is packed with vitamin A. Guacamole adds a burst of vitamin E that's great for your skin. Make extra for tomorrow's lunch.

PREPARATION TIME: 15 MINUTES ♥ **COOKING TIME:** 1 HOUR
SERVES 6

3 sweet potatoes, peeled,
    roughly cut into cubes
3 tablespoons coconut
    oil, melted, plus extra
    for greasing
1 cup quinoa, rinsed well
    and drained (or use
    cooked brown rice)
1½ cups vegetable stock
    (ideally homemade, but if
    store-bought ensure it is
    MSG free) or salted water
½ red onion, finely chopped
1 garlic clove, finely chopped
1 teaspoon ground cumin
½ teaspoon sweet paprika
1 teaspoon finely chopped
    coriander root
1 bird's eye chilli, seeded
    and chopped
¼ teaspoon sea salt
1 cup baby spinach
lime wedges, coriander sprigs
    and Healthy Guacamole
    (see page 217), to serve

Preheat the oven to 180°C and line a baking tray with baking paper.

Put the sweet potato in a large bowl and coat generously with the coconut oil. Spread out evenly on the lined tray and roast for 35–40 minutes or until tender and lightly caramelised. Set aside to cool slightly.

Meanwhile, combine the quinoa with the stock or water in a medium saucepan and bring to the boil over high heat. Reduce the heat and simmer, covered, for 15 minutes or until the quinoa has absorbed the liquid and each grain has a white spiral tail.

Grease a baking tray with coconut oil. Place the sweet potato in a large bowl and mash. Add the quinoa and mix gently using your hands, then mix in the onion, garlic, cumin, paprika, coriander root, chilli and salt. Shape the mixture into four or six burger patties and place them on the prepared tray. Bake for 20 minutes or until cooked to your liking.

Serve the burgers with the spinach, lime wedges, sprigs of coriander and the guacamole.

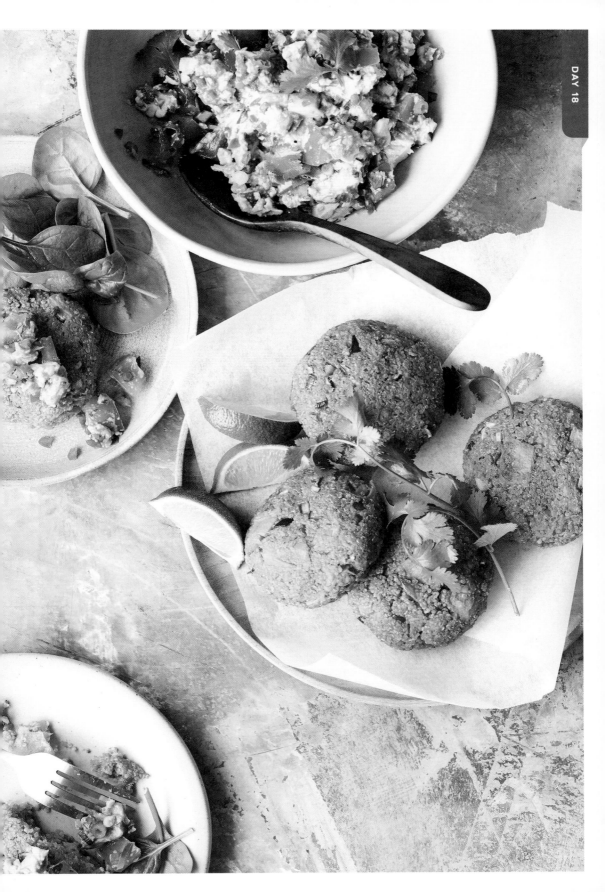

DAY 19

Are **cortisol** and **insulin** wreaking havoc on your skin?

Hormone fluctuations can be the culprit behind skin breakouts in teenagers and adults. Stress resulting from poor food choices, lack of sleep or the pressures of daily life increases cortisol and can be revealed through our skin. Over the years, I've seen wonderful improvements in skin health when people eat clean, low-sugar whole foods. De-stress by exercising – including walking or other cardio – or enjoying hobbies. Sleep for at least eight hours a night.

Foods that spike blood sugar levels often push the body to release extra insulin, increasing the production of cortisol and leading to skin breakouts, including rosacea. Reduce your sugar intake to natural sources only, such as low-sugar fruit and vegetables.

Skin-healthy foods include:

* **fish** – Filled with essential fatty acids, including omega-3, that reduce inflammation and assist with hormone balance. The best options are oily fish, including salmon, mackerel and sardines.
* **nuts** – Packed with zinc and selenium, minerals that are often deficient in people with acne. Eat them raw, activated or dry-roasted.
* **avocado** – Contains vitamin E, which gives skin a healthy glow. It's also packed with vitamin C, which reduces inflammation and naturally moisturises the skin from within.
* **fennel** – Full of vitamins, minerals and fibre. Fennel is a perfect skin cleanser, improves digestion and flushes out toxins.
* **artichokes** – Contain antioxidants and vitamin C, and are packed with fibre.
* **brown rice** – Contains vitamin B, protein and magnesium. Vitamin B is essential for making serotonin.
* **garlic** – Helps fight inflammation and is full of allicin, a compound that attacks harmful bacteria and viruses and supports the immune system.

* **broccoli** – A perfect skin-clearing food that contains health-building substances including the antioxidant vitamins A, B complex, C, E and K. These fight free radicals and help maintain skin luminosity.
* **alfalfa sprouts** – Packed with valuable skin-clearing nutrients, they also help fight inflammation.

TODAY'S ACTION

Today, include just one of the foods from the list above in your diet. I hope many of them are already on high rotation in your meals. When people ask what new skin regime you've started, just smile. Hydration and good nutrition is the reason your skin is glowing.

PRAWNS WITH MEXICAN CAULIFLOWER RICE

*Prawns are rich in selenium and iodine, two minerals that help the thyroid
to function effectively. Cauliflower is a powerful liver cleanser.*

PREPARATION TIME: 15 MINUTES, PLUS MARINATING TIME
COOKING TIME: 30 MINUTES ♥ SERVES 4

¾ teaspoon chilli powder

½ teaspoon ground cumin

1 teaspoon garlic powder

½ teaspoon sea salt,
plus extra to serve

¼ teaspoon chilli flakes

12 large green prawns,
peeled and deveined,
tails left intact

2 tablespoons extra virgin
olive oil

1 small onion, diced

1 red capsicum, seeded
and diced

3 garlic cloves, finely chopped

4 cups grated cauliflower

1 x 400 g tin diced tomatoes

2 tablespoons vegetable stock
(ideally homemade, but if
store-bought ensure it is
MSG free) or water

finely grated zest and juice
of 1 lime

diced avocado and coriander
sprigs, to serve

In a small bowl, mix the chilli powder, cumin, garlic powder, salt and chilli flakes.

In a separate bowl, toss the prawns with 1 tablespoon of olive oil and ½ teaspoon of the spice mixture until well coated. Cover and marinate in the fridge for 1 hour.

Heat a large frying pan over medium heat, add the prawns and fry for 2–3 minutes on each side. Remove from the pan and set aside.

Heat the remaining olive oil in the same pan over medium heat and sauté the onion and capsicum for 3–5 minutes or until they begin to soften. Add the garlic and cook for another minute. Add the grated cauliflower and remaining spice mixture, and stir until the cauliflower is well coated. Stir in the tomatoes and stock or water and bring to the boil, then reduce the heat to low and simmer, covered, for 5–10 minutes or until the cauliflower rice is cooked but still has some bite. Remove the lid and simmer for a few minutes to allow the excess liquid to evaporate.

Remove the pan from the heat and gently fold in the prawns, then add the lime zest and juice. Serve with diced avocado, coriander and a pinch of sea salt.

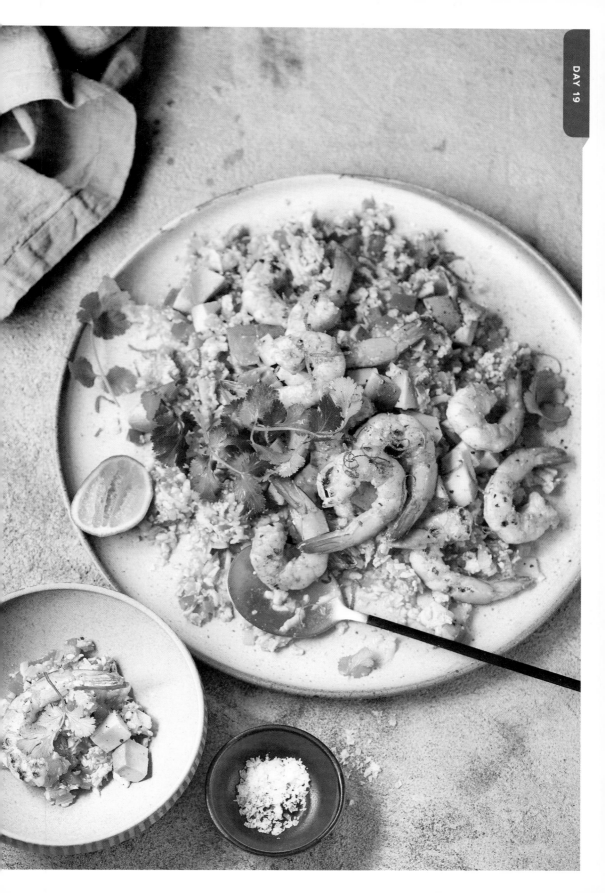

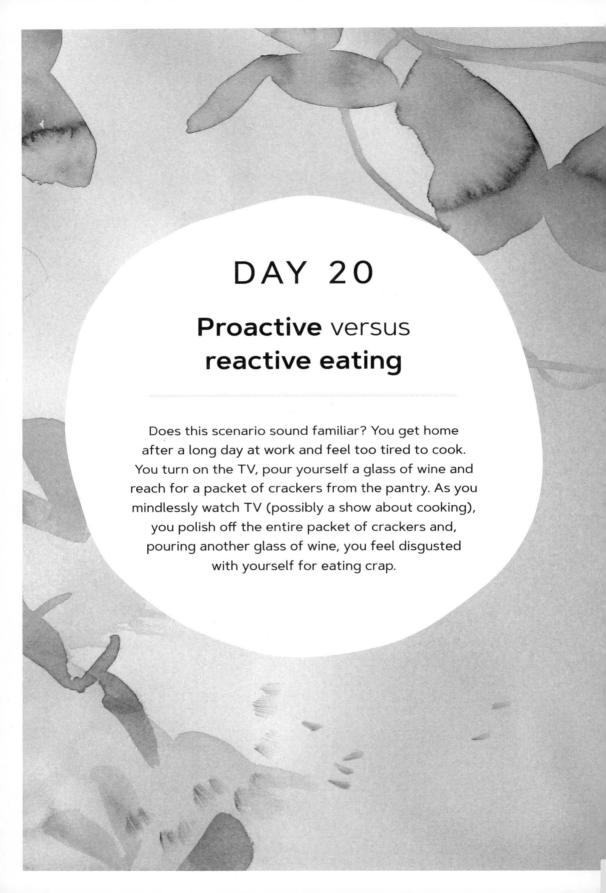

DAY 20

Proactive versus reactive eating

Does this scenario sound familiar? You get home after a long day at work and feel too tired to cook. You turn on the TV, pour yourself a glass of wine and reach for a packet of crackers from the pantry. As you mindlessly watch TV (possibly a show about cooking), you polish off the entire packet of crackers and, pouring another glass of wine, you feel disgusted with yourself for eating crap.

An hour later, you feel hungry again. Because you already feel like a failure, you eat more 'junk food' from the back of the pantry, food you bought for a special occasion. When you wake up the next morning, you're so appalled with yourself you skip breakfast. By lunchtime you're ravenous and heading to the vending machine for a chocolate bar or packet of chips. That was my story when I was a reactive eater.

Now, I'm a proactive eater. This means I plan, cook and prepare most of my meals and snacks. I know we're all busy and time-poor, but I urge you to examine the belief that you don't have time to plan your meals. If you don't make time for your health, you could miss out on other life opportunities, just because your body and brain aren't performing optimally. Physical and mental health is partly dependent on genetics, stress, toxic exposure and other factors we can't control. But we **can** control what we eat, and we can choose to eat fresh foods brimming with healthy nutrients.

I want you to think back to a time in your life when you achieved success. Did this success require planning? The same planning principles apply to healthy eating. During these 28 days, you're mastering these skills and creating habits for lasting physical and mental health.

TODAY'S ACTION

Plan each meal. Go shopping and be prepared. Eat well during the day so you don't come home starving. Ensure your pantry and refrigerator are filled with healthy food. Before eating, examine your plate. Can you improve the meal by adding more veggies or healthy fat?

Eating quickly has become the norm for most of us. Slow down, chew your food and savour the flavours — you will see instant improvement in your digestion.

GREEK LEMON CHICKEN

This recipe is a favourite with my children, particularly the zingy vitamin C-rich lemon.

PREPARATION TIME: 15 MINUTES, PLUS MARINATING TIME
COOKING TIME: 30 MINUTES ♥ SERVES 4

6 pieces preserved lemon rind
2 tablespoons lemon juice
2 garlic cloves, roughly
    chopped
1 teaspoon ground cumin
1 teaspoon sweet paprika
⅓ cup extra virgin olive oil,
    plus extra for drizzling
½ bird's eye chilli, seeded
½ bunch coriander,
    roughly chopped
4 x 150 g chicken breast fillets,
    skin on
green salad and lemon wedges,
    to serve

Process the preserved lemon, lemon juice, garlic, cumin, paprika, olive oil, chilli and coriander in a food processor for 2–3 minutes.

Using your thumb, gently lift the skin on each chicken breast and stuff the lemon mixture under it and around the entire breast. Place in a baking dish and sprinkle any remaining marinade over each breast, then cover and marinate in the fridge for at least 1 hour or overnight if possible.

Preheat the oven to 180°C.

Drizzle a little extra olive oil over the chicken breasts and roast for 30 minutes or until the juices run clear.

Serve the chicken with a fresh green salad and lemon wedges alongside.

TIPS: *This recipe also works well with white fish fillets, although the fish should be coated with the marinade rather than stuffing it under the skin. Another variation is to marinate 600 g chicken thighs on the bone in a mixture of chopped garlic, ground cumin, sweet paprika and 1 cup dried oregano. Your house will smell like a Greek kitchen.*

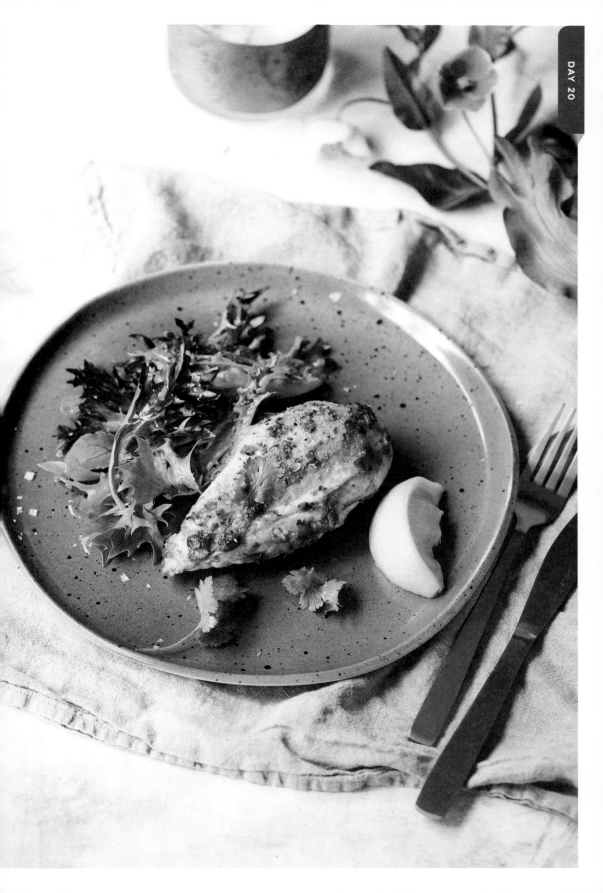

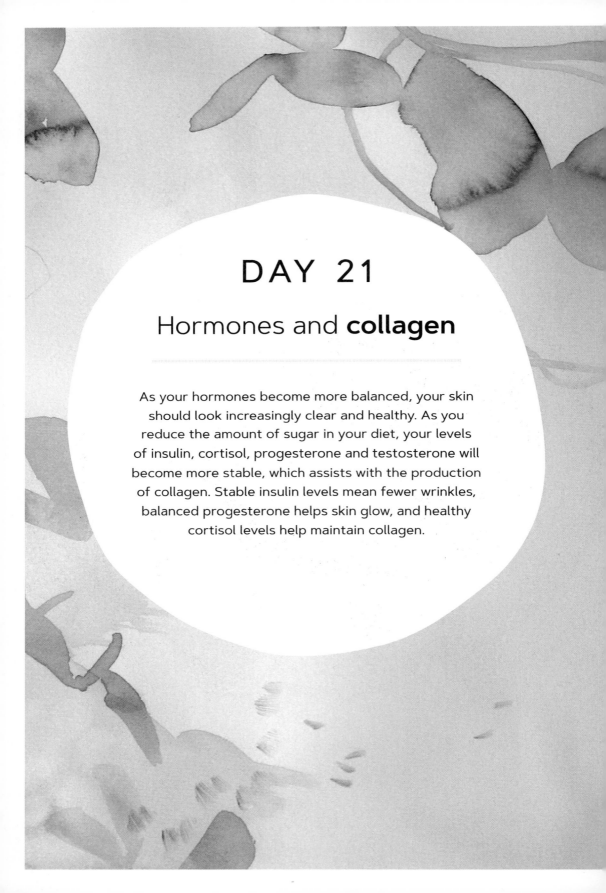

DAY 21

Hormones and **collagen**

As your hormones become more balanced, your skin should look increasingly clear and healthy. As you reduce the amount of sugar in your diet, your levels of insulin, cortisol, progesterone and testosterone will become more stable, which assists with the production of collagen. Stable insulin levels mean fewer wrinkles, balanced progesterone helps skin glow, and healthy cortisol levels help maintain collagen.

Collagen is part of the connective tissue in bones, skin and most of our organs. It affects the tightness of our wrinkles and supports every cell in the body. Without collagen, we look saggy. Collagen is affected by sugar, vitamin C, protein and phytonutrients. Too much sugar and the resulting insulin dysfunction leads to inflammation and oxidative stress, which produce advanced glycation end-products (AGEs). These AGEs damage collagen and elastin in the skin, which means our skin loses its elasticity and wrinkles form. To maintain collagen levels, the amount and quality of protein we eat is also important.

Vitamin C is essential for collagen synthesis. Excellent sources include broccoli, capsicum, kale, cabbage, cauliflower, brussels sprouts, spinach, silverbeet, snow peas, zucchini, fennel, asparagus, celery, tomatoes, lemons, papaya, kiwi fruit, rockmelon, oranges, grapefruit, lemons, limes, raspberries, strawberries, lettuce and parsley.

Other phytonutrients are also vital for skin health. Green tea has properties that help prevent the breakdown of collagen. (If you don't like the taste of green tea, mix it with flavours you do like, such as ginger or lemongrass.) Also helpful are the anthocyanidins found in dark-coloured red–blue berries and other fruits, such as blueberries, blackberries and raspberries. These phytonutrients help collagen fibres link together in a way that strengthens the matrix of connective tissue.

TODAY'S ACTION

Today, include foods that promote collagen. Enjoy a cup of green tea and a bowl of fresh blueberries. And remember that eating well, reducing stress and ensuring quality sleep all assist with maintaining collagen and skin health.

RED LENTIL SOUP

This tiny legume fills you up but not out. Red lentils are a great source of cholesterol-lowering fibre that also stabilises blood sugar levels. They are also packed full of B vitamins and magnesium.

PREPARATION TIME: 15 MINUTES ♥ COOKING TIME: 30 MINUTES
SERVES 4

2 tablespoons extra virgin
   olive oil
1 red onion, chopped
2 celery stalks, chopped
2 garlic cloves, finely chopped
1 leek, white part only,
   halved lengthways,
   washed and chopped
1 carrot, peeled if necessary,
   chopped
2 cups red lentils
1 sweet potato, peeled
   and chopped
2 litres vegetable or chicken
   stock (ideally homemade,
   but if store-bought ensure
   it is MSG free)
flat-leaf parsley or coriander
   leaves, to garnish

Heat the olive oil in a large heavy-based saucepan over medium heat. Add the onion, celery, garlic, leek and carrot and cook, stirring, for 5–6 minutes or until softened and lightly golden.

Wash and drain the lentils, then add to the pan with the sweet potato and stock. Bring just to the boil, then reduce the heat to low and simmer for 20 minutes or until the lentils and vegetables are soft.

Remove from the heat and allow to slightly cool, then purée in a blender or with a hand-held blender. Serve warm, garnished with parsley or coriander leaves.

TIP: *For an Asian influence, add 3 tablespoons of coconut milk and chilli and lemongrass to taste. Add the coconut milk right at the end after you have blended the soup and gently warm it through — but don't let it boil or it will curdle.*

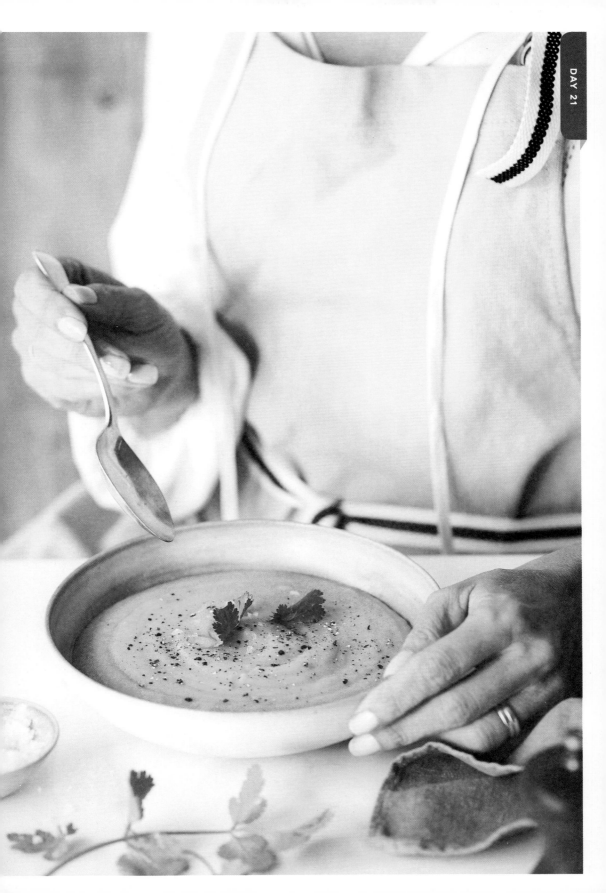

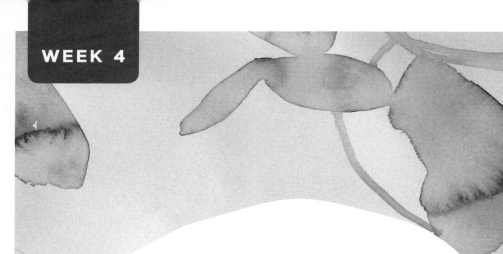

DAY 22

Is **MSG** messing with **your metabolism?**

When we eat good-quality protein foods, good fats and plenty of vegetables, we avoid most of the undesirable additives in processed foods. One additive to steer clear of is the flavour enhancer monosodium glutamate (MSG).

In one study, people who consumed
MSG had a higher prevalence of metabolic
syndrome, the collection of conditions that
increases the risk of diabetes. MSG has also
been associated with:

* fibromyalgia
* obesity
* fatty liver
* high insulin and blood sugar levels
* high cholesterol
* liver toxicity
* disturbances in the gut–brain connection
* neurological and brain damage.

MSG, listed on labels as E621, makes bland
foods tastier, which explains its popularity
among food manufacturers. The important
part of the molecule is glutamate, which can
be hidden under various names. Look out
for: glutamic acid (E620), glutamate (E620),
monopotassium glutamate (E622), calcium
glutamate (E623), monoammonium
glutamate (E624), magnesium glutamate
(E625), natrium glutamate, yeast extract,
anything hydrolysed, any hydrolysed protein,
calcium caseinate, sodium caseinate, yeast
food, yeast nutrient, autolysed yeast,
gelatine, textured protein, soy protein,
soy protein isolate, whey protein, whey
protein concentrate, whey protein isolate,
vetsin or ajinomoto.

TODAY'S ACTION

Today, look out for sources of MSG
and avoid it. This should be pretty
easy given you're eating whole foods
that don't come in a packet.

SIMPLE CHICKEN AND SWEET POTATO CHIPS

This is a far healthier version of good-old chicken and chips. And even the fussiest eater will love sweet potatoes prepared 'chip style'. A little chilli can be very beneficial — its thermogenic effect increases your metabolic rate.

PREPARATION TIME: 20 MINUTES, PLUS MARINATING TIME
COOKING TIME: 20 MINUTES ♥ SERVES 4

4 x 150 g skinless chicken
   breast fillets, cut into
   thin strips
2 bird's eye chillies, seeded
   and finely chopped
2 garlic cloves, crushed
finely grated zest and juice
   of 2 lemons
⅓ cup coconut oil
3 sweet potatoes, peeled and
   shredded into thin chips
1 tablespoon sweet paprika
sea salt and freshly ground
   black pepper
1 avocado, sliced
green salad, to serve

Place the chicken strips in a large bowl and toss with the chilli, garlic and lemon zest and juice. Cover and marinate in the fridge for as long as possible, but 30 minutes will do.

Melt 3 tablespoons of coconut oil in a large frying pan over medium heat, add the potato chips in batches and fry, turning them quickly so they do not burn, for 5–10 minutes or until golden brown. Remove to a plate lined with paper towel. Season if desired.

Meanwhile, heat the remaining coconut oil in a frying pan over medium heat. Add the chicken in batches and cook for 10 minutes or until brown on both sides and cooked through. Remove and cover to keep warm while you cook the remaining chicken. Season with the paprika, and salt and pepper to taste.

Serve immediately with the sweet potato chips, sliced avocado and a green salad. For salad dressings, see page 216.

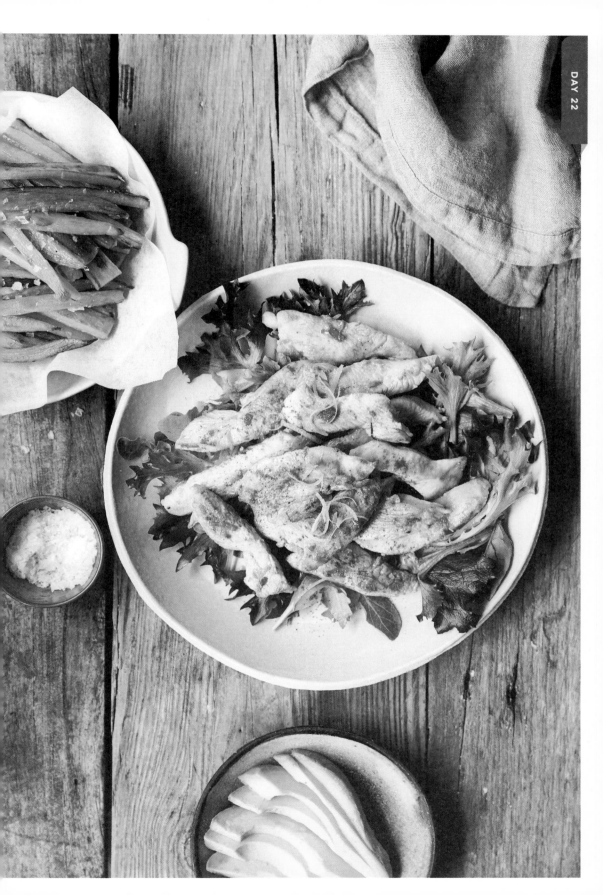

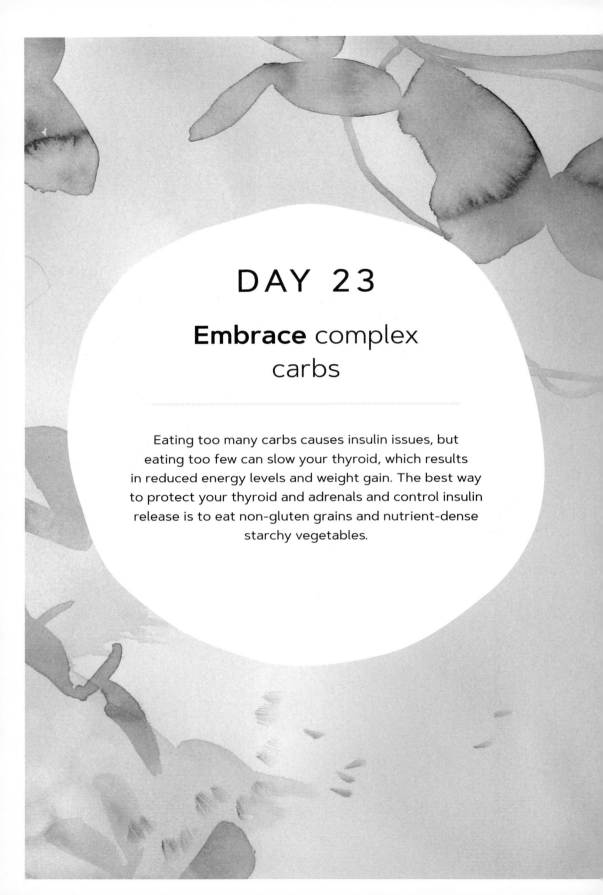

DAY 23

Embrace complex carbs

Eating too many carbs causes insulin issues, but eating too few can slow your thyroid, which results in reduced energy levels and weight gain. The best way to protect your thyroid and adrenals and control insulin release is to eat non-gluten grains and nutrient-dense starchy vegetables.

Not eating enough carbs can play havoc with your hormones, particularly cortisol and thyroid hormone. Carb-phobia is very real – the topic often comes up when I speak to groups of women. There's no need to be afraid of carbohydrates: say no to carb-phobia, but do get smart about which carbs you embrace. The best ones are the complex carbohydrates, the slow, gentle, smart and safe carbs in root vegetables such as sweet potatoes, beetroot, carrots, pumpkin and parsnips, and in brown rice, quinoa and buckwheat. Take a look at the starchy veggies in the shopping list on page 81. Other complex carbs include non-gluten grains that provide energy without spiking blood sugar levels or insulin.

When should you eat carbs on the rebalance? I'd like you to use food-combining principles at every meal (see pages 88–89). If you combine non-gluten grains and veggies, I prefer you to do this at breakfast or lunchtime rather than dinnertime. I'd rather you had a gluten-free carb during the day as a fuel supply. Good options include gluten-free buckwheat toast with avocado for breakfast or a veggie brown rice bowl for lunch.

TODAY'S ACTION

Today, embrace the complex carb. The amount you can eat will depend on your metabolism. Some people can eat mountains of carbs and never gain weight but others, like me, only have to look at carbs and the weight goes on. I consume low to moderate amounts of carbs to assist my adrenal and thyroid glands, which makes me a calmer, happier person.

BLACK BEAN CHILLI

There's a line in a song that children love to sing: 'Beans, beans, they're good for your heart.'
And it's true. The resistant starch in this zinc-packed bean won't cause a quick rise in blood
sugar levels. This phytonutrient-rich dish is high in fibre and iron.

PREPARATION TIME: 20 MINUTES
COOKING TIME: 1 HOUR 40 MINUTES ♥ SERVES 4

1 tablespoon extra virgin
    olive oil
2 red onions, finely chopped
2 garlic cloves, finely chopped
4 large carrots, peeled if
    necessary, chopped
2 large celery stalks, chopped
1 tablespoon chopped
    coriander, plus extra
    sprigs to serve
1 teaspoon cayenne pepper
½ teaspoon ground cumin
½ teaspoon smoked paprika
1 jalapeno chilli, finely chopped
    (optional)
1 x 400 g tin black beans,
    drained and rinsed
1 x 400 g tin red kidney beans,
    drained and rinsed
1 x 800 g tin diced tomatoes
700 g tomato passata
1 cup vegetable stock
1 small sweet potato, peeled
    and roughly chopped
2 teaspoons tomato paste
Healthy Guacamole
    (see page 217) and
    lime wedges, to serve

Heat the olive oil in a large heavy-based saucepan
over medium heat and add the onion, garlic, carrot and
celery. Stir well, then cook for 3–4 minutes or until the
onion is translucent. Stir in the coriander, cayenne,
cumin, paprika and chilli, if using, and cook for a further
1–2 minutes or until fragrant. Add the black beans,
kidney beans, diced tomatoes, tomato passata and
stock and mix well.

Pulse the sweet potato to rice-sized pieces in a food
processor and add to the pan. Bring to the boil, then
reduce the heat to low–medium and simmer, covered,
for 30 minutes. Stir in the tomato paste, then simmer
over low heat, covered, for 45 minutes–1 hour or until
cooked to your liking. (For maximum flavour, let it
simmer for up to 4 hours.)

Serve with the guacamole, lime wedges and
extra coriander.

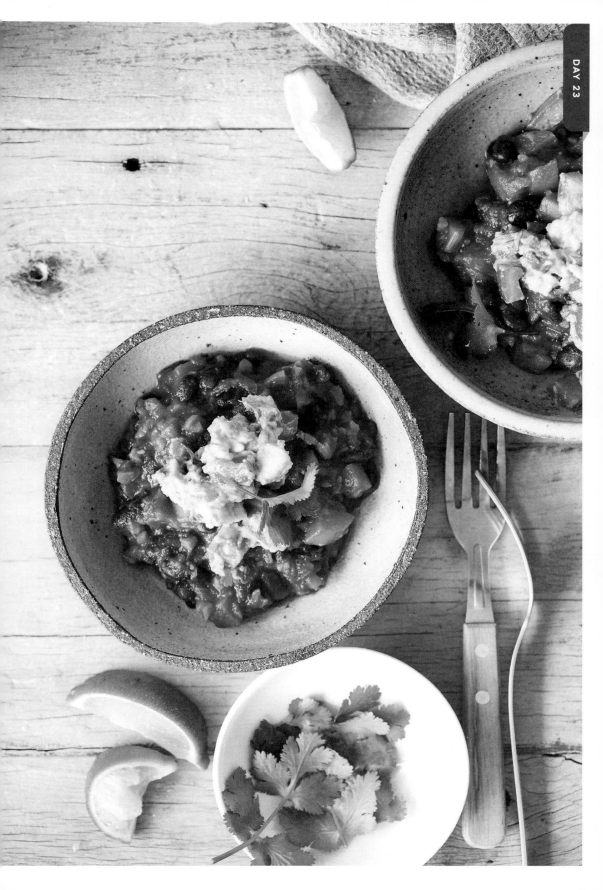

DAY 24

Hormones and gluten:
you be the judge

One aim of this rebalance is to help you discover how you feel when you eliminate particular foods from your diet. After that, you can make a choice about whether you reintroduce these foods based on that experience. I know gluten is a controversial topic but, in my experience, many clients who remove gluten from their diet feel better. Others remove gluten and don't feel a difference. Three-quarters of my clients who remove wheat, rye, oats and barley will later reintroduce rye, oats and barley but continue to avoid wheat. The choice is entirely yours.

Let me explain why I think gluten could be the cause of hormone imbalance in some people. When some people eat gluten, it creates an autoimmune reaction in the small intestine. The small projections called villi that line the small intestine become inflamed, reducing the surface area available for nutrient absorption. This condition is called coeliac disease and people who have it should avoid gluten completely.

Other people have a less serious gluten sensitivity, which can cause symptoms such as a bloated tummy, constipation or diarrhoea, or simply a vague feeling of 'unwellness'. The main issue is gliadin (see page 47), which is found in all gluten grains except gluten-free oats. Many people who suffer from gluten sensitivity are unaware of it. The symptoms can be vague and sometimes not felt in the gastrointestinal tract – brain fog or migraines, for example – which makes it hard to diagnose. Some people have a latent form of gluten sensitivity in which their immune system develops a response to gluten when triggered by acute stress, or a bacterial or viral infection, including food poisoning.

Gluten sensitivity can affect oestrogen and progesterone levels, particularly during menopause. In some cases, inflammation in the intestine causes more cortisol to be released, leading to weight gain and fatigue. Let's face it, if you're not absorbing nutrients very well, no wonder you feel exhausted! So why not see what happens when you remove wheat, rye, oats and barley from your diet.

TODAY'S ACTION

Because you've been following the rebalance, you're already experimenting with a gluten-free life. How do you feel? Have you noticed any differences? Be a label detective with gluten-free products. Remember that a gluten-free stamp on a packet doesn't necessarily mean it's healthy. It could easily contain fillers and sugar, so investigate further.

GLUTEN-FREE FOODS

Gluten is often added to soup mixes, sauces, soy sauce, lollies, salad dressings and low-fat foods. According to the Food Standards Australia New Zealand code, foods labelled gluten-free must not contain any detectable gluten. Ingredients derived from gluten-containing grains must be declared on the food label, and foods labelled as 'low gluten' must have less than 200 parts per million of gluten. Non-gluten grains include buckwheat, quinoa, amaranth, rice and millet.

THAI CHICKEN BURGERS

Herbs and spices make this chicken burger a winner. Natural antibiotic garlic provides bite while coriander brings a pungent, citrus flavour.

PREPARATION TIME: 10 MINUTES ♥ COOKING TIME: 15 MINUTES
SERVES 4

700 g chicken mince,
    preferably thigh (see tip)
3 garlic cloves, finely chopped
½ cup finely chopped coriander
3 golden shallots,
    finely chopped
3 teaspoons fish sauce
½ teaspoon sea salt
½ teaspoon freshly ground
    black pepper
2 teaspoons finely chopped
    bird's eye chilli (optional)
2 teaspoons coconut oil
mixed salad and lime wedges,
    to serve

Place the chicken, garlic, coriander, shallot, fish sauce, salt, pepper and chilli, if using, in a bowl and mix together well with your hands. Form the mixture into four even patties.

Heat a non-stick frying pan over medium heat. Rub both sides of each patty with a little of the coconut oil and cook for about 8 minutes on the first side and 5 minutes on the other side, or until the patties are firm to the touch and cooked through.

Serve with a salad and lime wedges alongside.

TIP: *Chicken thighs are higher in iron than chicken breasts.*

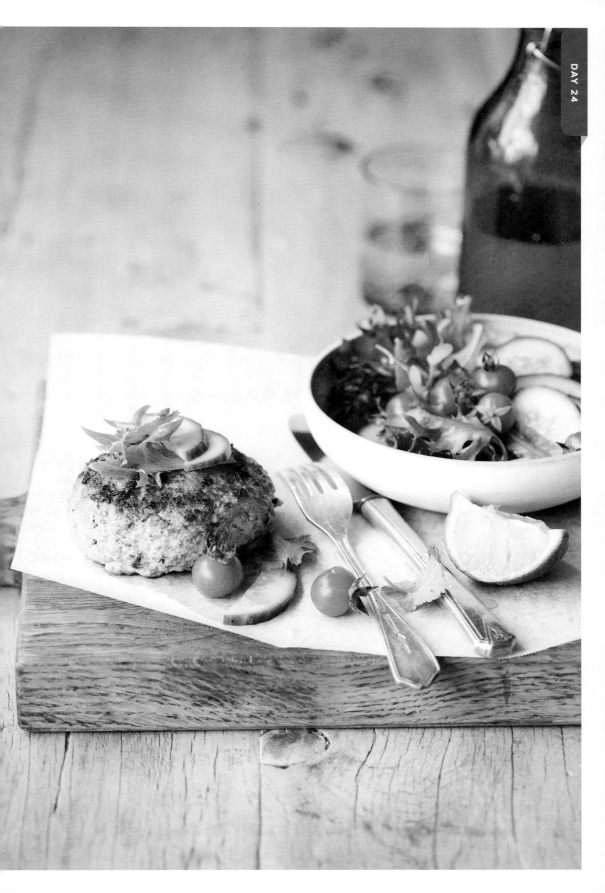

DAY 25

Insulin and **soft drinks**

Soft drinks and other sugary drinks are bad for us in so many ways. My advice is just don't drink them. For one, they're packed full of sugar. And you already know the negative effects of sugar on your body, from weight gain to increased risk of type 2 diabetes. But in my view, even drinks made with artificial sweeteners should be avoided. There's limited research in this area, and the results depend on the type of artificial sweetener used, but one theory suggests that because artificial sweeteners are significantly sweeter than regular sugar, they activate our genetically programmed preference for sweet tastes.

When ingested, they trick our metabolism into thinking sugar is on its way. This may cause our body to pump out insulin, which triggers the body to lay down more belly fat. (In addition to soft drinks, artificial sweeteners can be found in yoghurts, confectionery, jellies, fruit drinks, cordials, milk-based puddings, sports drinks, energy drinks and weight-management products.)

Another possible effect they have is to increase cravings for carbohydrates. One study found that mice fed artificial sweeteners underwent changes in gut bacteria and had increased blood sugar levels. There's also a view that artificial sweeteners confuse our metabolism so we burn fewer calories every day. Even though the effect on humans isn't definitive, I advise my clients to avoid both types of drinks – sugary and artificially sugary.

The Harvard School of Public Health has highlighted an alarming collection of statistics on the connection between soft drinks and disease. I'll highlight just a couple of them for you. According to Harvard, the Nurses' Health Study 'found that women who drank more than two servings of sugary beverage each day had a 40 per cent higher risk of heart attack or death from heart disease than women who rarely drank sugary beverages'. And 'The nurses who said they had one or more servings a day of a sugar-sweetened soft drink or fruit punch were twice as likely to have developed type 2 diabetes during the study than those who rarely had these beverages'.

As mentioned earlier, soft drinks affect magnesium levels in the body. Dark-coloured soft drinks in particular contain phosphates that bind with magnesium in the digestive tract. Rather than being absorbed by the body, the magnesium goes straight through the system unused. When we eat refined sugar, this also makes the body excrete magnesium through the kidneys. The more sugar we consume, the more likely we are to be deficient in magnesium. Caffeine also releases more magnesium through the kidneys.

The logical conclusion? Just drink water.

TODAY'S ACTION

Drink water, every day. For variety, you can also try sparkling water, teas or iced herbal tea with fruit slices. For a hint of sweetness, add a pinch of stevia, a natural sweetener.

THYME CHICKEN WITH ROAST VEGETABLES

Thyme is a completely underrated herb. For one, it's packed with vitamins A and C. For many years, thyme was used in the treatment of colds, flu and respiratory problems.

PREPARATION TIME: 15 MINUTES ♥ COOKING TIME: 20 MINUTES
SERVES 4

4 x 150 g skinless chicken
  breast fillets
⅓ cup extra virgin olive oil,
  plus extra if needed
1 teaspoon sea salt, plus extra
  to taste
finely grated zest of 2 lemons
1 bunch thyme, leaves picked
3 baby eggplants or 1 medium
  eggplant, cut into 2 cm
  cubes or 5 mm-thick rounds
¼ cauliflower, separated
  into florets
2 sweet potatoes, peeled and
  cut into 2 cm cubes
3 zucchini, cut into 5 mm-thick
  rounds
200 g baby rocket
freshly ground black pepper

Preheat the oven to 180°C and line two baking trays with baking paper.

Place the chicken breasts on one of the lined trays. Drizzle with half the olive oil, and scatter over the salt, lemon zest and half the thyme leaves.

Arrange the eggplant, cauliflower, sweet potato and zucchini on the second tray (or put them all on one large tray if you have one). Coat generously with the remaining olive oil and salt to taste, and scatter over the remaining thyme leaves.

Roast the chicken and vegetables for 20 minutes or until cooked through (it will depend on the thickness of the chicken fillets). Serve with the rocket and finish with a good grinding of pepper.

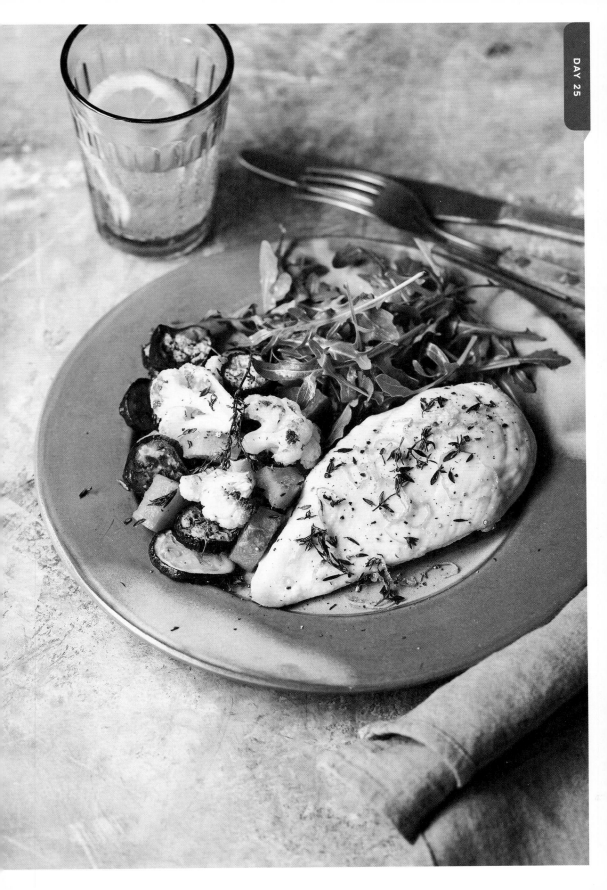

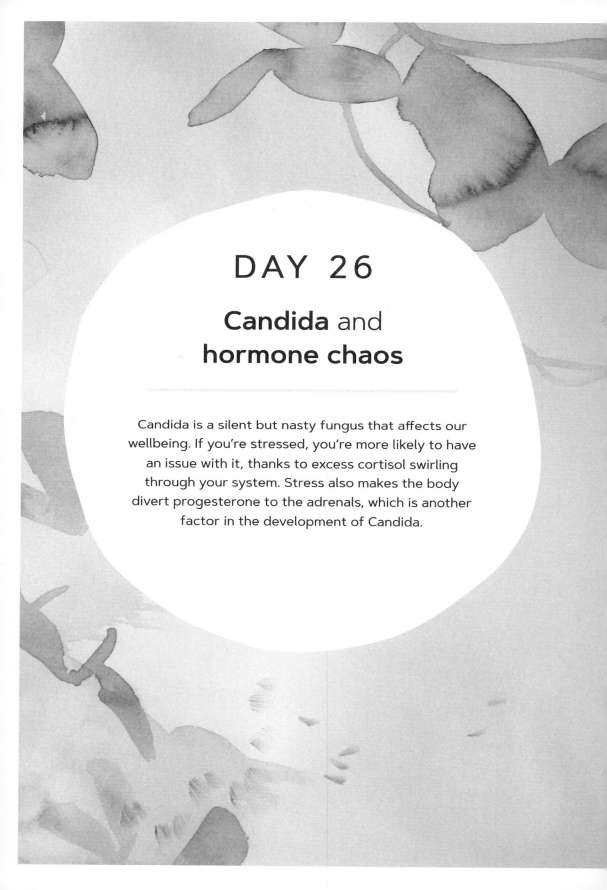

DAY 26

Candida and hormone chaos

Candida is a silent but nasty fungus that affects our wellbeing. If you're stressed, you're more likely to have an issue with it, thanks to excess cortisol swirling through your system. Stress also makes the body divert progesterone to the adrenals, which is another factor in the development of Candida.

Among our gut microbiota is a yeast fungus called Candida albicans. It can live there quite happily until it doesn't. Candida infections affect the skin and mucous membranes, and one factor affecting their trajectory is hormones – particularly oestrogen and progesterone – which cause it to spread beyond the digestive tract. When Candida overgrowth occurs, it can be in the uncomfortable form of vaginal thrush or nail and foot fungus.

Two common promoters of Candida infections are birth-control pills and a high-sugar diet. Candida loves sugar, particularly blood-sugar spikes and crashes. Candida is more common among diabetics and affects insulin resistance.

Diets high in sugar can lead to insulin resistance and cortisol overload, which dampens the production of calming progesterone. As oestrogen levels increase, Candida can spread like wildfire from stress and a sugar-packed liver.

As discussed earlier, 90 per cent of serotonin is synthesised in the gut, so it makes sense that overgrowth of Candida in the gut can disrupt serotonin levels by interfering with normal gut functions and upsetting the normal balance of the microbiome. Chronic stress increases cortisol levels and reduces the number of good bacteria in the gut. It's an invitation for opportunistic bacteria to invade, causing inflammation, fungal infections and Candida overgrowth.

TODAY'S ACTION

By embarking on this rebalance, you've taken steps to reduce stress, eat whole foods and reduce sugars, so you should already be experiencing a reduction in Candida-related symptoms such as bloating, cravings and brain fog.

Be aware that as Candida dies off, it can create a short-term reaction. When it happened to me it felt like being hit by the world's worst flu: I experienced headaches, achy joints and tiredness. I don't collapse easily and it made me realise just how toxic my life had been. If this happens to you, rest assured it soon passes. Increase your good intestinal flora with a probiotic supplement, so they help push Candida out. (I'm not a supplement pusher but I do believe that a quality fish oil and a probiotic are a worthwhile investment in your health.) Clean eating will keep your gut flora healthy and strong. Eat probiotic foods such as kimchi, sauerkraut, yoghurt and fresh garlic.

LEMON TARRAGON PRAWN SKEWERS

Tarragon is the herb of choice for the French. With a slight smell of aniseed, it is abundant in phytonutrients, manganese, iron and calcium.

PREPARATION TIME: 15 MINUTES, PLUS MARINATING TIME (OPTIONAL)
COOKING TIME: 15 MINUTES ♥ SERVES 4

1 lemon, cut into 8 wedges
24 medium green prawns,
    peeled and deveined,
    tails left intact
olive oil, for cooking
80 g mixed salad leaves

LEMON TARRAGON DRESSING

⅓ cup lemon juice
3 teaspoons olive oil
1 tablespoon finely
    chopped tarragon
2 teaspoons dijon mustard

If you are using bamboo skewers, soak them in water for about 5 minutes so they don't burn during cooking. You will need eight skewers for this recipe.

Thread a lemon wedge and three prawns onto each skewer.

To make the lemon tarragon dressing, combine all the ingredients in a glass jar, seal tightly and shake well. If time permits, drizzle half the dressing over the prawns and marinate in the fridge for 1–2 hours.

Heat a barbecue grill plate or large chargrill pan over high heat. Drizzle over some olive oil and grill the skewers, in batches if necessary, for 2–3 minutes on each side or until just cooked.

Serve the prawn skewers with the salad leaves and the remaining dressing.

TIP: *This recipe also works well with scallops or firm fish fillets instead of the prawns.*

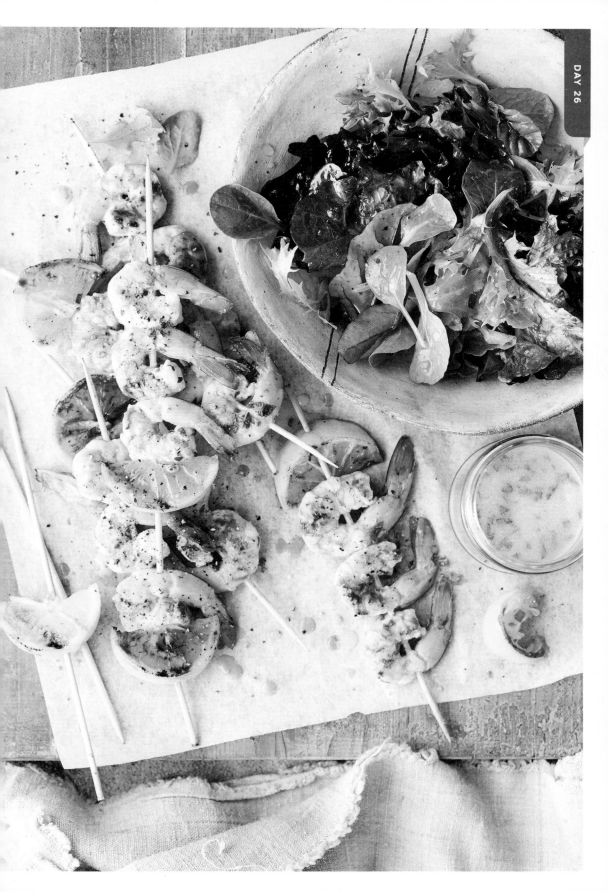

DAY 27

Hormones and chronic **inflammation**

Inflammation is implicated in many conditions, from psoriasis to obesity, heart disease, osteoporosis, arthritis and Alzheimer's disease. Inflammation isn't all bad news, particularly when it's related to an allergy or infection. In this instance, the body releases pro-inflammatory compounds to relieve the stress or damage until it returns to normal. But if it doesn't return to its resting state, chronic inflammation rears its head.

Inflammation can be caused by excess weight; a diet high in sugar, processed food and unhealthy fats; excess alcohol; lack of exercise; stress; smoking; and prolonged exposure to pollution. The release of too much cortisol can cause an unhealthy inflammatory imbalance. Stress increases cortisol levels, with flow-on effects to other hormones. When cortisol is too high it takes more insulin to drive glucose into cells. High cortisol and high insulin are the reason our waist expands, because instead of burning fat, the body stores it. But when cortisol is in balance, it's a wonderful anti-inflammatory. And while we can't control every trigger for inflammation, we can control what we eat and how we manage stress. The reason some 75-year-olds are still doing crosswords while others are struggling with their memory could come down to inflammation.

Dr Richard Johnson, head of Renal Diseases and Hypertension at the University of Colorado and author of *The Sugar Fix* and *The Fat Switch*, argues that humans aren't designed to eat large amounts of refined sugar, cereal and bread. When we consume too many sugars and carbs, it upsets our hormone signalling, making us feel hungry and crave sweet foods. Sugar promotes inflammation. Dietary carbohydrates, including fructose and other processed sugars, starches, celluloses and gums, lead to excess body fat and obesity. One study found that drinking sugar-sweetened beverages regularly was associated with an increased risk of death from cardiovascular disease. A recent study found that high-fructose corn syrup, a common sweetener in the United States, is a contributor to asthma. The easiest way to avoid these foods is to think twice before stuffing them in.

TODAY'S ACTION

If you find yourself reaching for a refined carb, remind yourself they offer only empty calories that strip the body of vitamins and minerals. You feel hungrier after eating them because they interfere with hormone signalling and because your body needs nutrient-dense foods. Processed foods can also slow your metabolism and cause inflammation. How do you feel? Do you have less joint pain and fewer headaches? This means you're tackling inflammation.

LENTIL, BEETROOT AND HERB SALAD

There is so much I love about this salad, from the beetroot with betalains that promote liver detoxification, to the protein- and iron-rich lentils. The abundant fibre is excellent for removing toxins.

PREPARATION TIME: 20 MINUTES ♥ COOKING TIME: 20 MINUTES
SERVES 4

4 beetroot, peeled and cut
   into bite-sized cubes
2 x 400 g tins lentils,
   drained and rinsed
4 spring onions, thinly sliced
1 cup mint leaves
1 cup baby rocket
sea salt and freshly ground
   black pepper

GINGER DRESSING
1 tablespoon grated ginger
½ cup extra virgin olive oil
2 teaspoons dijon mustard
1 tablespoon apple
   cider vinegar

Place the beetroot in a medium saucepan, cover with water and bring to the boil. Reduce the heat and simmer, covered, for 15 minutes or until tender. Drain and set aside to cool.

Meanwhile, combine the lentils, spring onion, mint and rocket in a bowl. Gently fold in the beetroot and season to taste.

To make the dressing, place all the ingredients in a small food processor and blend until smooth. Gently toss through the salad and serve.

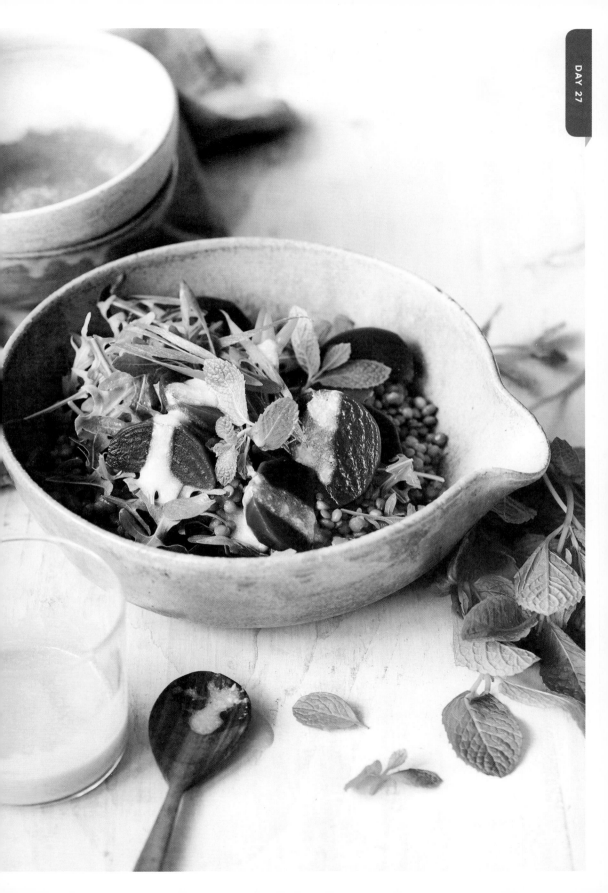

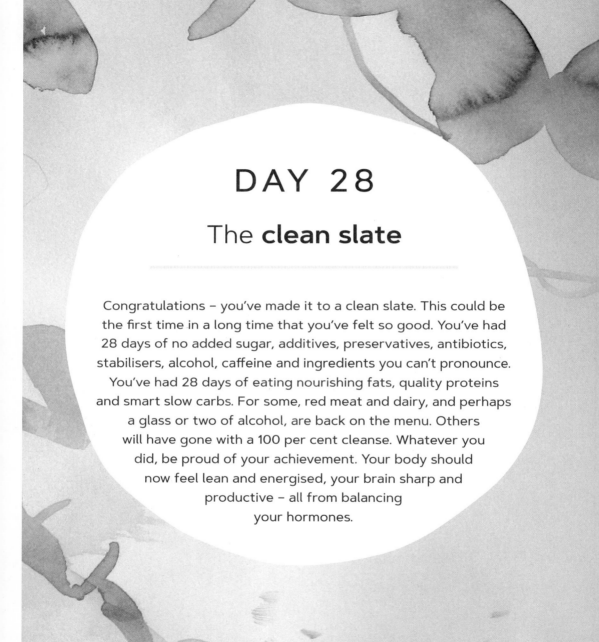

DAY 28

The **clean slate**

Congratulations – you've made it to a clean slate. This could be the first time in a long time that you've felt so good. You've had 28 days of no added sugar, additives, preservatives, antibiotics, stabilisers, alcohol, caffeine and ingredients you can't pronounce. You've had 28 days of eating nourishing fats, quality proteins and smart slow carbs. For some, red meat and dairy, and perhaps a glass or two of alcohol, are back on the menu. Others will have gone with a 100 per cent cleanse. Whatever you did, be proud of your achievement. Your body should now feel lean and energised, your brain sharp and productive – all from balancing your hormones.

What happens now that you've completed the rebalance? When I tell clients they can stop following the plan and reintroduce the foods they've crowded out, most pause, stare at me and declare, 'Why would I do that when I feel so good? Imagine if I'd known how to manage my mood, energy and hormonal swings years ago? Imagine what I might have achieved?'

For more on reintroducing foods, see page 212. But for now, here are some general points. If you followed the rebalance to the letter, you eliminated added sugar, red meat, dairy, gluten, alcohol, excessive caffeine and processed foods. If you reintroduce any of these foods, do it slowly and reintroduce one item at a time. That way you can know if a reaction – such as headache, brain fog, sleepiness, bloating, puffiness, weight gain, constipation, diarrhoea, eczema, joint issues or muscle aches – is due to that food.

It's difficult to grasp unless you see, feel and experience this change. Wait for one week until you reintroduce another food. Trust me on this. Many people reintroduce foods too quickly and waste the benefits of their clean slate. When you finally discover the culprit behind your zapped energy, weight gain and moodiness, you'll be thankful. Reactions are your way of diagnosing food sensitivities. You don't necessarily need a lab report.

You'll notice that we don't reintroduce processed foods, foods with added sugar, excessive caffeine and alcohol. When I'm not following the rebalance, I drink one or two coffees a day with a splash of A2 milk and one glass of wine three or four nights a week. I consider this to be 'choosing my poison'. Feel free to say this when offered a piece of birthday cake at the office or a glass of red wine at dinner. Choose your poison. I can happily live without processed foods and I very rarely eat anything with added sugar. When you become used to it, savoury flavours will be the norm and you'll lose the cravings for sugar that once ruled your moods and energy.

TODAY'S ACTION

Because you look and feel amazing, many friends and family will be in awe of you. But others will want to sabotage your efforts with snide comments like, 'Jane doesn't drink any more. Boring!'. Or 'Charlotte's no fun because she doesn't eat pizza.' Or 'Peter doesn't eat out any more so let's stop inviting him.' Don't allow saboteurs to enter your health zone. Most people want to be at their best but find change scary. You can and will eat out, drink wine and, if you choose, eat pizza – perhaps gluten-free. Be clear with your intentions, your progress and your vision of who you want to be.

If you can, try intermittent fasting this evening. If not, enjoy fantastic fish parcels.

FANTASTIC FISH PARCELS WITH SPICED FENNEL

Parcels make food fun! The fennel adds flavour, anti-inflammatory qualities and lovely flavonoids such as rutin and quercetin. Rutin helps the body use vitamin C and maintain collagen levels.

PREPARATION TIME: 15 MINUTES ♥ **COOKING TIME:** 30 MINUTES
SERVES 4

pinch of finely grated
    lemon zest
juice of 1 lemon, plus extra
    wedges to serve
2 garlic cloves, crushed
2 teaspoons grated ginger
4 chervil sprigs, plus extra
    to serve
1 teaspoon extra virgin olive oil
1 fennel bulb, trimmed and
    thinly sliced
2 teaspoons Moroccan
    spice blend
4 x 150 g white fish fillets
    (such as snapper, ling
    or barramundi), skin
    and bones removed
green salad or steamed
    broccoli tossed with garlic
    and extra virgin olive oil,
    to serve

Preheat the oven to 180°C.

Combine the lemon zest and juice, garlic, ginger and chervil in a bowl.

Heat the olive oil in a small frying pan over medium heat, and sauté the fennel with the Moroccan spice blend for about 5 minutes.

Tear off four large squares of baking paper. Divide the fennel mixture among the paper squares and place a fish fillet on top. Drizzle over the lemon mixture, then gather the corners of the baking paper to create a parcel, securing tightly with kitchen string, seam-side up.

Place the parcels on a baking tray and bake for 20–25 minutes or until the fish is cooked through. Let them stand for 5 minutes, then top with extra chervil. Serve with a green salad or steamed broccoli, and lemon wedges.

TIP: *A Thai spice mix also works well here.*

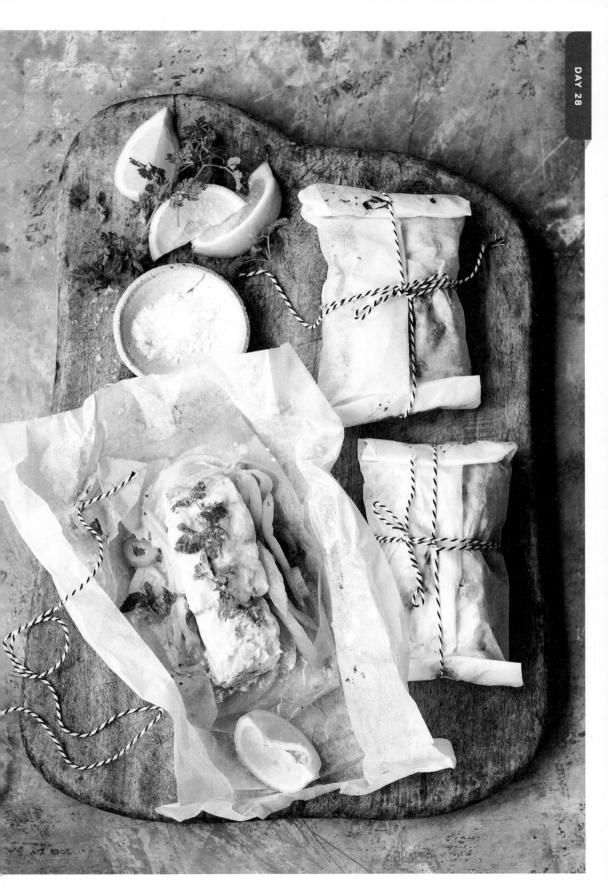

LIFE BEYOND THE REBALANCE

Once you've completed the rebalance, you can start to reintroduce foods each week and make notes about how they make you feel. That will help you determine the kind of eating pattern you can maintain into the future to keep your health, energy and happiness at their optimum levels. Notice how your body reacts if you stop the food-combining principles.

* **WEEK 5:** *Rye, oats and barley*

This week, reintroduce rye, oats and barley but remain wheat-free. This will help you narrow down what is the reason for any tummy upsets you may have experienced in the past.

Make a note of how you react to these foods (you can keep notes on your phone for easy tracking). If it turns out you can tolerate rye, oats and barley, then great. There's no need to avoid a food if you don't react to it.

* **WEEK 6:** *Wheat*

Reintroduce wheat, including pasta, bread and cereal. Fads or trends should never be the reason you exclude particular types of food from your diet. You should only cut out a particular food if your body has a negative reaction to eating it. When eating wheat, don't go overboard. Limit your intake to two pieces of quality bread, a serve of cereal or a bowl of pasta each day.

* **WEEK 7:** *Dairy*

Reintroduce A2 or organic milk. If you can tolerate dairy, great, but I strongly suggest sticking with A2 or organic milk rather than returning to standard milk. Full-fat is fine.

* **WEEK 8:** *Beef and lamb*

If you haven't done so already, reintroduce beef and lamb. One reaction you may observe is slower bowel movements. This is particularly the case as we age, because our system produces fewer digestive enzymes. When eating red meat, include bitter foods such as rocket or endive to stimulate digestion. Where possible, choose grass-fed, pasture-fed or organic meats.

* **WEEK 9:** *Break the rules!*

Did you discover what foods work best for you? Write down what worked and what didn't. Later, if you feel sluggish, repeat the principles of the rebalance, even if only for one week. As outlined earlier, break one rule at a time and leave a few days before breaking another rule. For example, combine fruit and yoghurt. Watch what happens to your tummy, mood and weight. If you feel fine, break the next rule. Eat fish with rice or chicken with lentils. Do you feel sluggish or bloated, or energised and vibrant?

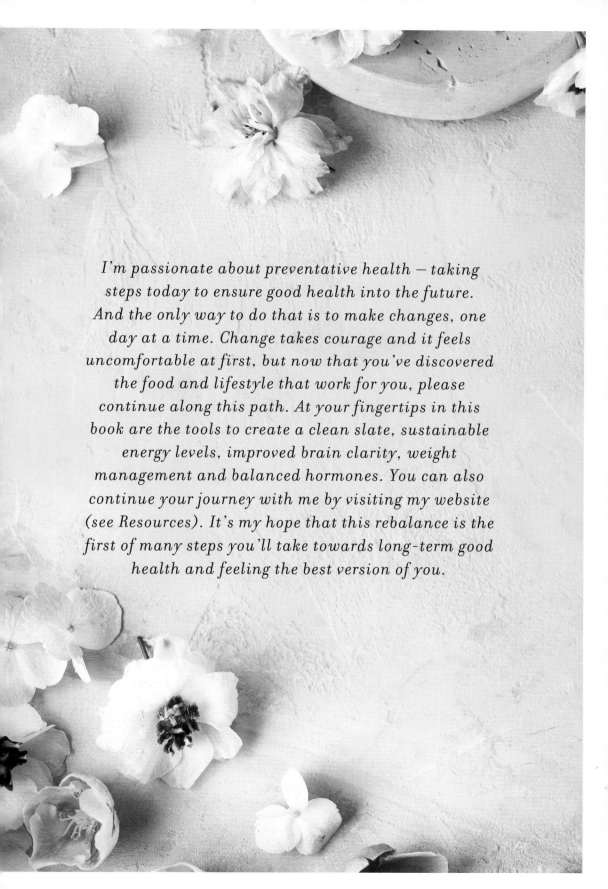

I'm passionate about preventative health — taking steps today to ensure good health into the future. And the only way to do that is to make changes, one day at a time. Change takes courage and it feels uncomfortable at first, but now that you've discovered the food and lifestyle that work for you, please continue along this path. At your fingertips in this book are the tools to create a clean slate, sustainable energy levels, improved brain clarity, weight management and balanced hormones. You can also continue your journey with me by visiting my website (see Resources). It's my hope that this rebalance is the first of many steps you'll take towards long-term good health and feeling the best version of you.

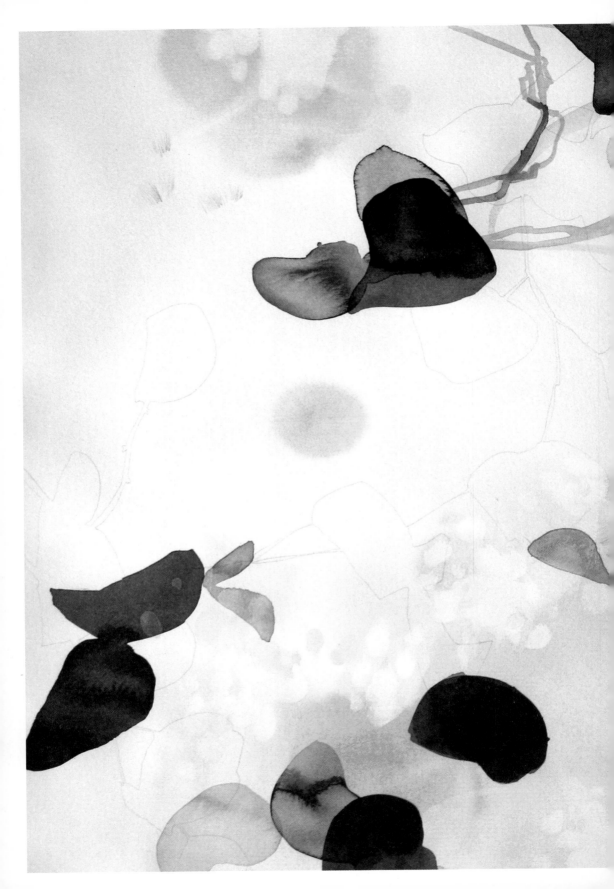

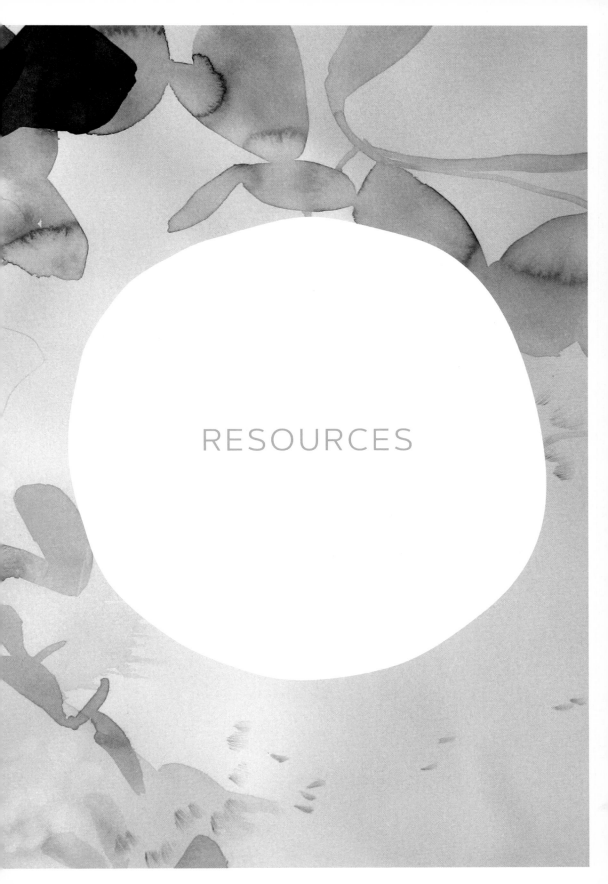

RESOURCES

DRESSINGS

Don't be hesitant to use dressings that contain quality fats. They are a great accompaniment to salads, protein/veggie meals and grain/veggie meals.

CHERMOULA DRESSING

1 tablespoon sweet paprika
½ teaspoon cayenne pepper
6 garlic cloves, finely chopped
½ cup lemon juice
3 tablespoons finely chopped
    flat-leaf parsley
3 tablespoons finely chopped coriander
½ cup extra virgin olive oil
sea salt and freshly ground black pepper

Place all the ingredients in a large bowl and whisk to combine well. Allow to sit for 15 minutes before serving.

GINGER LIME DRESSING

3 tablespoons lime juice
3 tablespoons tamari
2 tablespoons finely chopped spring onion
2 tablespoons grated ginger
2 tablespoons toasted sesame oil
2 tablespoons extra virgin olive oil

Place all the ingredients in a small blender and blend until well combined.

LEMON DRESSING

3 tablespoons extra virgin olive oil
2 tablespoons lemon juice
2 teaspoons finely chopped garlic
1 teaspoon chopped thyme or tarragon
½ teaspoon mustard powder
½ teaspoon finely grated lemon zest
sea salt and freshly ground black pepper

Place all the ingredients in a glass jar, seal tightly and shake vigorously for about 30 seconds.

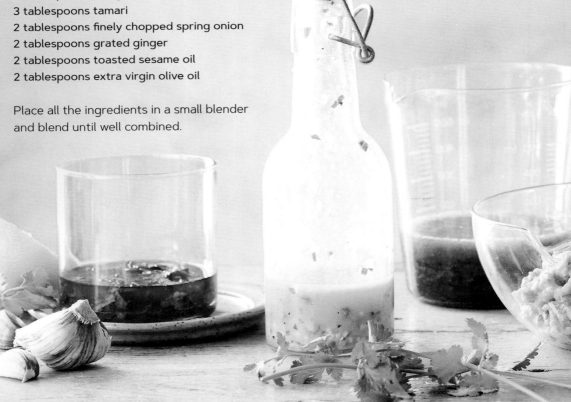

HERBIE SAUCE

juice of 1 lemon
juice of ½ lime
3 tablespoons chopped flat-leaf parsley
1 tablespoon finely chopped basil
1 tablespoon finely chopped oregano
1 tablespoon finely chopped dill
2 garlic cloves, finely chopped
1 bulb spring onion, finely chopped
2 tablespoons extra virgin olive oil
sea salt

Place all the ingredients in a glass jar, seal tightly and shake well, or purée in a blender.

SMOOTH AVOCADO VINAIGRETTE

1 ripe avocado
2 garlic cloves, finely chopped
juice of 1 lime
2 teaspoons extra virgin olive oil
1 bird's eye chilli, seeded and chopped
sea salt and freshly ground black pepper

Place all the ingredients in a blender or food processor and purée until creamy, adding a little water to thin if needed.

TIP: *For a variation, add 3–5 chopped basil leaves, 1 teaspoon dulse or kelp flakes and 2–3 chopped spring onions.*

HEALTHY GUACAMOLE

2 ripe avocados, mashed
4 spring onions, thinly sliced
1 large tomato, finely diced
2 garlic cloves, crushed
½ jalapeno chilli, finely chopped
⅓ cup lime juice
3 tablespoons chopped coriander
½ teaspoon sea salt

Place all the ingredients in a bowl and mash with a fork. For a smoother consistency, pulse in a food processor or blender.

TIP: *To ripen avocados, leave them overnight in a brown paper bag with a ripe banana.*

PORTION SIZE GUIDE

You won't always have scales or measuring cups on you, but you will have your eyes, so learn how to work out portion sizes by sight.

Food type	Amount per day	By eye	Notes
Protein foods	Multiply your goal weight by 1.5 or, if athletic, by 2. For example, a woman aiming to weigh 70 kg can eat 105 g of protein per day. An athletic man aiming to weigh 100 kg can eat 200 g of protein per day. A 150 g serve of fish contains about 20 g protein.	The size of your palm	This is a generous portion. You can eat less, but I don't want you to feel hungry an hour later. Protein foods keep you feeling full.
Non-starchy vegetables	No limit	-	-
Starchy vegetables	½–2 cups	The size of your fist	For optimum weight loss, eat starchy carbs at lunch and avoid at dinner.
Fruit	1–2 pieces	The size of your fist	-
Good fats and oils ＊ Extra virgin oil ＊ Avocado ＊ Nuts and seeds	⅓ cup ¼–½ 30–40 g	A very generous splash Half the size of your palm A closed fistful	Men can eat more
Non-gluten grains	½–1 cup	A closed fistful	Men can eat more. For optimum weight loss, no more than one serving per day.

SUGAR: THE OTHER SUSPECTS

OTHER NAMES FOR SUGARS

* Agave nectar
* Agave syrup
* Barley malt
* Beet sugar
* Brown rice solids
* Brown sugar
* Buttered syrup
* Cane juice
* Cane juice crystals
* Cane sugar
* Carob syrup
* Confectioners' sugar
* Corn sugar
* Corn sweetener
* Corn syrup
* Corn syrup solids

* Crystallised fructose
* Date sugar
* Dextran
* Dextrose
* Diastase
* Diastatic malt
* Evaporated cane juice
* Fructose
* Fruit juice
* Fruit juice concentrate
* Glucose
* Glucose solids
* Golden sugar
* Golden syrup
* Grape juice concentrate
* Grape sugar

* High-fructose corn syrup
* Honey
* Invert sugar
* Lactose
* Malt
* Maltodextrin
* Maltose
* Maple syrup
* Molasses
* Raw sugar
* Refiners' syrup
* Sorghum syrup
* Sucanat
* Sucrose
* Turbinado sugar

TRACKING YOUR PROGRESS

I don't think a weigh-in each week on a set of scales is the best measure of progress because our weight can fluctuate, particularly in response to hormones.

But after my clients demanded it, I gave in and have scales in my clinic that provide bio-impedance analysis (BIA).

This measures:

* **Cellular hydration** – Cellular hydration is important for many biochemical processes. It helps the body deliver and absorb nutrients, and eliminate toxins, and assists in tissue function in the body and brain. The greater the hydration, the easier it is to lose weight.
* **Percentage of body fat** – Too little or too much fat can affect our hormones, weight and self-esteem. See the table below for how percentage body fat relates to health.
* **Weight** – I emphasise to clients that scales are only a physical measure and don't reflect our value or worth.

Other measures can give you an indication of your progress, including:

* **Waist circumference** – This is an indicator of health risk from excess fat around the waist. A circumference of 102 cm or more for men or 88 cm or more for women is associated with type 2 diabetes, heart disease and high blood pressure.
* **Visceral fat** – This is the fat you can't see, that is stored in the abdomen, around the liver, pancreas and intestines. It can play an important part in hormone function and is associated with type 2 diabetes. I see many 'slender rusters' – people who

	Body condition	Aged 20–39	Aged 40–59	Aged 60–79
WEIGHT MEASUREMENTS – PERCENTAGE BODY FAT				
Men	Underweight	less than 8	less than 13	less than 13
	Normal	8–20	13–22	13–25
	Overweight	20–25	22–28	25–30
	Obese	more than 25	more than 28	more than 30
Women	Underweight	less than 21	less than 23	less than 24
	Normal	21–33	23–34	24–36
	Overweight	33–39	34–40	36–42
	Obese	more than 39	more than 40	more than 42

are slim on the outside but 'rusting' on the inside. This is particularly the case for white-collar men over the age of 40, who often have a slim appearance but dangerous inflammatory fat on the inside. Visceral fat is measured by an MRI, bio-impedance analysis or a DEXA scan.

* **Blood tests** – These can indicate whether your health is on the way up or silently going downhill. It doesn't tell the entire story, but it does offer a useful report card. I work alongside GPs and medical specialists.

Ask your doctor to request the following blood tests:

* a full blood count
* iron studies (including ferritin levels)
* cholesterol studies
* thyroid-stimulating hormone (TSH)
* urinary iodine
* if you suspect you have thyroid issues, test for thyroid antibodies free T3 and T4
* vitamin D
* fasting insulin
* fasting glucose (this is not a glucose tolerance test or GTT)
* vitamin B12
* leptin
* the inflammatory markers C-reactive protein (CRP) and erythrocyte sedimentation rate (ESR)
* reproductive hormones (your GP will tell you at which part of your cycle to be tested); hormones measured include oestradiol, progesterone and DHEA
* cortisol levels – this can be tested in blood, saliva or urine.

The best nutrients are in real whole foods, and my philosophy is food first before supplements. But there can be a time and a place for additional support. Supplements should not be taken without consulting your GP or a qualified nutritionist.

NUTRIENTS FOR **GENERAL HORMONAL HEALTH**

Nutrient or supplement	Benefit	Foods found in	Notes
Co-enzyme Q10 (CoQ10)	∗ Increases energy production in cells ∗ Alleviates fatigue and muscle/joint pain ∗ Potent antioxidant	Grass-fed beef, herring, trout, peanuts, sesame seeds, pistachios, broccoli, cauliflower	Statins (cholesterol-lowering medication) can lower CoQ10 levels. Consult your GP.
Omega-3 fatty acids (EPA and DHA)	∗ Anti-inflammatory ∗ Repairs nerves ∗ Balances hormones	Cold-water fish (salmon, trout), walnuts, pecans, most nuts and seeds, olive oil, walnut oil	-
Vitamin B complex	∗ Essential for production of energy, serotonin and red blood cells ∗ Helps maintain brain and adrenal health ∗ Balances mood	Salmon, trout, lamb, mushrooms, hazelnuts, walnuts	-
Vitamin D3	∗ Involved in hormone balance and immune regulation ∗ Assists with calcium absorption into bone ∗ May improve immunity, assist in weight loss and lessen risk factors for cancer and depression	Grass-fed butter, ghee, cod liver oil, salmon, mackerel, sardines, milk, egg yolk	Time in sunshine is required for the body to make its own vitamin D

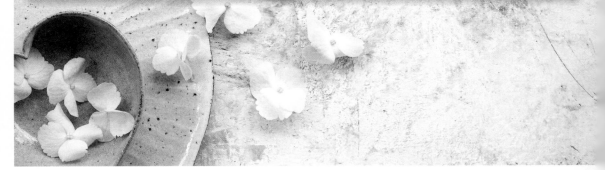

NUTRIENTS FOR **GENERAL HORMONAL HEALTH**

Nutrient or supplement	Benefit	Foods found in	Notes
Probiotics	* Promote healthy gut flora for digestion and elimination	Probiotic foods: kimchi, coconut kefir, sauerkraut, cow's, sheep's and goat's yoghurt, pickles, tempeh, miso Prebiotic foods (which support the gut flora): garlic, leek, onion	There are many strains of probiotics. Consult a qualified practitioner.
Magnesium	* Known as the great calmer * Relaxes muscles and nerve spasm * Relieves constipation * Assists sleep * Prevents insulin resistance * Supports thyroid function	Pumpkin seeds, yoghurt, kefir, almonds, black beans, avocado, dark leafy vegetables	Up to 75 per cent of Australians are estimated to be magnesium-deficient
Zinc	* Powerful antioxidant * Boosts immunity and testosterone levels	Grass-fed beef, lamb, kefir or yoghurt, chickpeas, pumpkin seeds, cashews, chicken, mushrooms, spinach	Often deficient in people with inflammatory conditions
Vitamin C	* Helps with inflammation * Powerful antioxidant * Improves collagen synthesis – keeps skin youthful * Essential for iron absorption * Super supporter of the adrenal glands	Sweet potato, green leafy vegetables, broccoli, beetroot, capsicum, garlic, radishes, parsley, grapefruit, lemon, limes, kiwi fruit	-

NUTRIENTS FOR **CORTISOL HEALTH**

Nutrient or supplement	Benefit	Foods found in	Notes
Herbs and fungi	* May help reduce stress	Astragalus root, cordyceps, licorice, ginseng, holy basil and ashwagandha	-
Vitamins	* May help reduce stress	A quality multivitamin, vitamins C, B (especially B6 and B5)	-
Vitamin B12	Assists with: * nerve and brain function * creation of red blood cells * energy	Sardines, tuna, salmon, grass-fed beef, lamb, eggs, shiitake mushrooms, nutritional yeast	Vegans and vegetarians can be deficient

NUTRIENTS FOR **SEROTONIN HEALTH**

Nutrient or supplement	Benefit	Foods found in	Notes
St John's Wort	* Elevates mood	-	-
Iron bisglycinate	* Supports energy * Increases protein digestion and nutrient absorption	Lentils, black beans, spirulina, grass-fed beef, spinach, sardines, pistachios. After the rebalance, raisins and dark chocolate	Iron is the vital component of haemoglobin, which transports oxygen in the blood. Iron in this form is easier on the stomach.
5-hydroxytrypto-phan (5-HTP)	* Precursor to serotonin * Assists with emotional stability * Reduces sleep disturbance	Cheese, chicken, turkey, milk, spirulina, eggs, wild-caught fish, grass-fed beef, lamb, legumes, nuts and seeds, sweet potato	-
S-adenosylmethi-onine (SAME)	* Assists with serotonin and dopamine production * Improves mental clarity	-	-
L-glutamine	* Helps with gut repair, especially the small intestine lining	Animal foods, spinach, kale, parsley, eggs, beetroot, carrots, collagen powder, bone broth	-

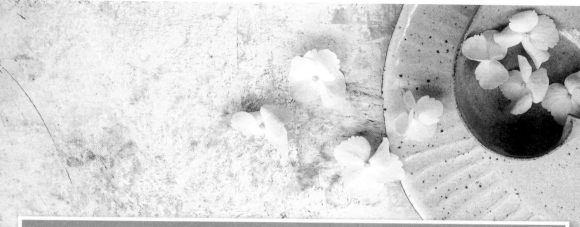

NUTRIENTS FOR **THYROID HORMONE HEALTH**

Nutrient or supplement	Benefit	Foods found in	Notes
Herbs	* Assist with thyroid health	Ashwagandha, holy basil and rhodiola	-
Vitamin A	* Helps with the integrity of gut lining * Supports the immune system * Assists with the assimilation of other nutrients	Butter, ghee, eggs, carrots, sweet potato, kale, spinach, broccoli, pumpkin	Without fat in the diet, we don't absorb vitamins A, D, E and K (the fat-soluble vitamins)
Selenium	* Potent antioxidant * Helps convert inactive thyroid hormone (T4) to the active form (T3)	Nuts and seeds, silverbeet, turnips, garlic	-
Iodine	Assists with: * thyroid function * metabolism * brain development in babies * fertility * the immune system	Seafood, especially seaweed, nori rolls, dulse flakes	-

NUTRIENTS FOR **INSULIN AND LEPTIN** HEALTH

Nutrient or supplement	Benefit	Foods found in	Notes
Herbs	* May support insulin balance * Powerful anti-inflammatory and insulin regulators * Regulate glucose and lipid metabolism that affects weight	Ginseng, spirulina, licorice, berberine, bitter melon	-
Alpha-lipoic acid (ALA)	* Enhances insulin sensitivity * Detoxifies heavy metals * Reduces inflammation * Antioxidant	Red meat, tomatoes, beetroot, carrots, green vegetables (especially broccoli, spinach, brussels sprouts, peas)	-
Manganese	Assists with: * blood sugar regulation * energy metabolism * thyroid function	Pecans, walnuts, turnips, rhubarb, thyme, cinnamon, turmeric	-
Fibre	Assists with: * blood sugar regulation * lowering cholesterol * weight loss	Flaxseeds, chia seeds, legumes, vegetables, konjac root	-

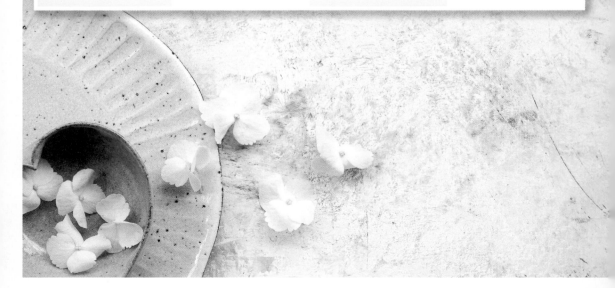

NUTRIENTS FOR **OESTROGEN** HEALTH

Nutrient or supplement	Benefit	Foods found in	Notes
Liver-cleansing herbs and foods	* Support liver health	St Mary thistle, cabbage, kale, cauliflower, broccoli, brussels sprouts	Treatment depends on whether oestrogen is low or high. If the liver is healthy, it naturally detoxifies excess oestrogen.
Other herbs	Assist with: * metabolic function * hormone regulation * PMS * inflammation	Evening primrose oil	–

NUTRIENTS FOR **TESTOSTERONE** HEALTH

Vitamins C and D3, zinc, magnesium	* Support testosterone metabolism	See pages 222–223 for foods containing these nutrients	

FOR MORE INFORMATION, comments and feedback from others on the rebalance, join my private Facebook group, Healthy Hormone Rebalance.

To continue your hormone rebalance journey, and for more information on nutrients, food and supplements, visit us at ahealthyview.com/healthyhormonerebalance.

REFERENCES

PART 1: WHAT'S HAPPENING WITH YOUR HORMONES?

Hormones and weight

Page 16   Chronically high insulin levels …: Christiane Northrup, *The Wisdom of Menopause: Creating Physical and Emotional Health During the Change*, Bantam Books, New York, 2011, p. 516.

What causes hormone chaos?

Page 19   It contributes to insulin resistance: Robert A. Rizza, Lawrence J. Mandarino & John E. Gerich, 'Cortisol-induced insulin resistance in man: impaired suppression of glucose production and stimulation of glucose utilization due to a postreceptor defect of insulin action', *Journal of Clinical Endocrinology & Metabolism*, 1982, vol. 54, no. 1, pp. 131–38.

Page 19   In a study at Ohio State University …: Janice K. Kiecolt-Glaser et al., 'Daily stressors, past depression, and metabolic responses to high-fat meals: a novel path to obesity', *Biological Psychiatry*, 2015, vol. 77, no. 7, pp. 653–60.

PART 2: ARE YOUR HORMONES IN HARMONY?

Cortisol: the stress hormone

Page 28   They decrease levels of the happy hormone …: P.J. Cowen, 'Cortisol, serotonin and depression: all stressed out?' *British Journal of Psychiatry*, 2002, vol. 180, no. 2, pp. 99–100.

Page 29   In a long-term study …: Sanjay R. Patel & Frank B. Hu, 'Short sleep duration and weight gain: a systematic review', *Obesity* (Silver Spring), 2008, vol. 16, no. 3, pp. 643–53.

Page 29   Vitamin B6 and an amino acid …: P.H. Mehta & R.A. Josephs, 'Testosterone and cortisol jointly regulate dominance: evidence for a dual-hormone hypothesis', *Hormones and Behavior*, 2010, vol. 58, no. 5, pp. 898–906.

Page 30   When we're stressed, we're more likely …: Mary F. Dallman et al., 'Chronic stress and obesity: A new view of "comfort food"', *Proceedings of the National Academy of Sciences*, 2003, vol. 100, no. 20, pp. 11696–701.

Insulin: the fat-storage controller

Page 34   But too much insulin can block …: M. Kellerer et al., 'Insulin inhibits leptin receptor signalling in HEK293 cells at the level of janus kinase-2: a potential mechanism for hyperinsulinaemia-associated leptin resistance', *Diabetologia*, 2001, vol. 44, no. 9, pp. 1125–32.

Page 34   When insulin levels spike …: George L. Blackburn, Vay Liang W. Go & John Milner (eds), *Nutritional Oncology*, 2nd edn, Elsevier, Amsterdam, 2006, pp. 186.

Page 34   At the time of writing …: ' "Metabolic reproductive syndrome" proposed as new name for PCOS', *Healio: Endocrine Today*, 7 July 2016, healio. com/endocrinology/reproduction-androgen-disorders/news/online/%7B5203193f-8ab8-44f3-9f1e-111a565cac62%7D/metabolic-reproductive-syndrome-proposed-as-new-name-for-pcos

Page 35   In one study, overall insulin sensitivity …: Josiane L. Broussard et al., 'Impaired insulin signaling in human adipocytes after experimental sleep restriction: a randomized, crossover study', *Annals of Internal Medicine*, 2012, vol. 157, no. 8, pp. 549–57.

Page 35   Fat cells need sleep …: Amanda Gardner, 'Too little sleep may fuel insulin resistance', CNN, 16 October 2012, edition.cnn.com/2012/10/15/health/sleep-insulin-resistance

Page 37   Those diagnosed with metabolic syndrome …: Kyong Park et al., 'Oxidative stress and insulin resistance: the Coronary Artery Risk Development in Young Adults study', *Diabetes Care*, 2009, vol. 32, no. 7, pp. 1302–307.

Page 37   Sugar consumption is also implicated …: F.W. Danby, 'Nutrition and aging skin: sugar and glycation', *Clinics in Dermatology*, 2010, vol. 28, no. 4, pp. 409–11.

Thyroid: the queen of metabolism

Page 38   More than 70 per cent of those with thyroid problems …: Gregory A. Brent, 'Environmental exposures and autoimmune thyroid disease', *Thyroid*, 2010, vol. 20, no. 7, pp. 755–61.

Page 39   It can be triggered by a number of factors …: C. Sategna-Guidetti et al., 'Prevalence of thyroid disorders in untreated adult celiac disease patients and effect of gluten withdrawal: an Italian multicenter study', *American Journal of Gastroenterology*, 2001, vol. 96, no. 3, pp. 751–57.

Page 39   … environmental toxins – bisphenol A (BPA) and …: 'Environmental agents trigger autoimmune thyroid disease', *Medscape Medical News from the American Thyroid Association (ATA) Paul W. Mamula*, PhD, Spring 2010 Meeting, 20 May 2010, presented May 15, 2010.

Page 41   When inflammatory foods such as gluten

and dairy ...: L. Bartalena et al., 'Relationship of the increased serum interleukin-6 concentration to changes of thyroid function in nonthyroidal illness', *Journal of Endocrinological Investigation*, 1994, vol. 17, no. 4, pp. 269–74.

Page 41   If you have a thyroid issue ...: Chin Lye Ch'ng, M. Keston Jones & Jeremy G.C. Kingham, 'Celiac disease and autoimmune thyroid disease', *Clinical Medicine and Research*, 2007, vol. 5, no. 3, pp. 184–92; C. Sategna-Guidetti et al., 'Autoimmune thyroid diseases and coeliac disease', *European Journal of Gastroenterology and Hepatology*, 1998, vol. 10, no. 11, pp. 927–32.

Page 41   It attacks organs associated ...: A. Fasano, 'Leaky gut and autoimmune diseases', *Clinical Reviews in Allergy and Immunology*, 2012, vol. 42, no. 1, pp. 71–78.

Page 42   Despite cutting out gluten ...: S.W. Spaulding et al., 'Effect of caloric restriction and dietary composition of serum T3 and reverse T3 in man', *Journal of Clinical Endocrinology & Metabolism*, 1976, vol. 42, no. 1, pp. 197–200.

Page 42   Even though most thyroid problems ...: T. Mizokami et al., 'Stress and thyroid autoimmunity', *Thyroid*, 2004, vol. 14, no. 12, pp. 1047–55.

Serotonin: the happy hormone and neurotransmitter

Page 46   ... one in seven Australians ...: 'Facts & figures about mental health and mood disorders', Black Dog Institute, n.d., blackdoginstitute.org.au/docs/default-source/factsheets/facts_figures.pdf?sfvrsn=8

Page 46   Even though research is in its infancy ...: Dr. Siri Carpenter, 'That gut feeling', *Monitor on Psychology*, 2012, vol. 43, no. 8, p. 50.

Page 47   More than 90 per cent of serotonin ...: Sarah Dash et al., 'The gut microbiome and diet in psychiatry: focus on depression', *Current Opinion in Psychiatry*, 2015, vol. 28, no. 1, pp. 1–6.

Page 47   Preliminary findings suggest a link ...: Xuguang Guo et al., 'Sweetened beverages, coffee, and tea and depression risk among older US adults', *PLOS ONE*, 2014, vol. 9, no. 4, article no. e94715.

Page 47   This triggers zonulin ...: Karin de Punder & Leo Pruimboom, 'The dietary intake of wheat and other cereal grains and their role in inflammation', *Nutrients*, 2013, vol. 5, no. 3, pp. 771–87.

Page 47   As health advocate Michael Pollan says ...: Michael Pollan, *Food Rules: An Eater's Manual*, Penguin, New York, 2009, p. 7.

Page 48   The indicators of iron deficiency ...: Leonid B. Trost, Wilma F. Bergfeld & Ellen Calogeras, 'The diagnosis and treatment of iron deficiency and its potential relationship to hair loss', *Journal of the American Academy of Dermatology*, 2006, vol. 54, no. 5, pp. 824–44.

Page 48   The link between the gut, brain and stress ...: Simon R. Knowles, Elizabeth A. Nelson & Enzo A. Palombo, 'Investigating the role of perceived stress on bacterial flora activity and salivary cortisol secretion: a possible mechanism underlying susceptibility to illness', *Biological Psychology*, 2008, vol. 77, no. 2, pp. 132–37.

Page 50   If not, they can lead ...: Alec Coppen & Christina Bolander-Gouaille, 'Treatment of depression: time to consider folic acid and vitamin B12', *Journal of Psychopharmacology*, 2005, vol. 19, no. 1, pp. 59–65.

Testosterone: the hormone of vitality

Page 53   Drinking in the evening ...: Eliza Van Reen et al., 'Does timing of alcohol administration affect sleep?', *Sleep*, 2011, vol. 34, no. 2, pp. 195–205.

Page 53   Men who drink excessive alcohol ...: Mary A. Emanuele & Nicholas V. Emanuele, 'Alcohol's effects on male reproduction', *Alcohol Health and Research World*, 1998, vol. 22, no. 3, pp. 195–201.

Page 53   Too little sleep alters metabolism ...: Guglielmo Beccuti & Silvana Pannain, 'Sleep and obesity', *Current Opinion in Clinical Nutrition and Metabolic Care*, 2011, vol. 14, no. 4, pp. 402–12.

Page 53   In one study, a group of healthy older men ...: Plamen D. Penev, 'Association between sleep and morning testosterone levels in older men', *Sleep*, 2007, vol. 30, no. 4, pp. 427–32.

Page 53   In another study, lack of sleep ...: Rachel Leproult & Eve Van Cauter, 'Effect of 1 week of sleep restriction on testosterone levels in young healthy men', *JAMA*, 2011, vol. 305, no. 21, pp. 2173–74. doi:10.1001/jama.2011.710

Page 53   Zinc (40 mg a day) is also important ...: A. Netter, R. Hartoma & K. Nahoul, 'Effect of zinc administration on plasma testosterone, dihydrotestosterone, and sperm count', *Archives of Andrology*, 1981, vol. 7, no. 1, pp. 69–73.

Page 53   In one study, overweight men ...: S. Pilz et al., 'Effect of vitamin D supplementation on testosterone levels in men', *Hormone and Metabolic Research*, 2011, vol. 43, no. 3, pp. 223–25.

Page 54   ... which suggested leptin resistance ...: Joseph R. Vasselli et al., 'Dietary components in the development of leptin resistance', *Advances in Nutrition*, 2013, vol. 4, no. 2, pp. 164–75.

Page 55   Nearly 40 per cent of obese men ...: P. Dandona & M.T. Rosenberg, 'A practical guide to male hypogonadism in the primary care setting', *International Journal of Clinical Practice*, 2010, vol. 64, no. 6, pp. 682–96.

Page 55   Cholesterol medication also affects ...: C. Mary Schooling et al., 'The effect of statins on testosterone in men and women: a systematic review and meta-analysis of randomized controlled trials', *BMC Medicine*, 2013, vol. 11, no. 57.

Leptin: the hunger hormone

Page 56   When working well, leptin ...: Chang Hee Jung CH & Min-Seon Kim, 'Molecular mechanisms of central leptin resistance in obesity', *Archives of Pharmacological Research*, 2013, vol. 36, no. 2, pp. 201–207.

Page 57   Studies reveal a link between sleep ...: Karine Spiegel et al., 'Leptin levels are dependent on sleep duration: relationships with sympathovagal balance, carbohydrate regulation, cortisol, and thyrotropin', *Journal of Clinical Endocrinology and Metabolism*, 2004, vol. 89, no. 11, pp. 5762–71.

Page 57   A summary of 36 sleep studies ...: Sanjay R. Patel & Frank B. Hu, 'Short sleep duration and weight gain: a systematic review', *Obesity (Silver Spring)*, 2008, vol. 16, no. 3, pp. 643–53.

Page 57   In one study, young men who slept ...: Karine Spiegel et al., 'Brief communication: Sleep curtailment in healthy young men is associated with decreased leptin levels, elevated ghrelin levels, and increased hunger and appetite', *Annals of Internal Medicine*, 2004, vol. 141, no. 11, pp. 846–50.

Page 58   Rats fed a 60 per cent fructose diet ...: Alexandra Shapiro et al., 'Fructose-induced leptin resistance exacerbates weight gain in response to subsequent high-fat feeding', *American Journal of Physiology – Regulatory, Integrative and Comparative Physiology*, 2008, vol. 295, no. 5, pp. R1370–75.

Page 60   ... and this would assist her in achieving ...: Janne E Reseland et al., 'Effect of long-term changes in diet and exercise on plasma leptin concentrations', *American Journal of Clinical Nutrition*, 2001, vol. 73, no. 2, pp. 240–45.

Oestrogen: the protective hormone

Page 62   If too high, it can cause weight gain ...: National Cancer Institute, 'Genetics of breast and gynecologic cancers', National Institutes of Health (US), 11 May 2017, cancer.gov/types/breast/hp/breast-ovarian-genetics-pdq

Page 65   Have you been diagnosed with type 2 diabetes?: Gineet Kaure Jasuja et al., 'Circulating estrone levels are associated prospectively with

diabetes risk in men of the Framingham Heart Study', *Diabetes Care*, 2013, vol. 36, pp. 2591–96.

Page 65   In one study, women who drank ...: Francine Grodstein et al., 'Relation of female infertility to consumption of caffeinated beverages', *American Journal of Epidemiology*, 1993, vol. 137, no. 12, pp. 1353–60.

Page 65   ... research suggests that the chemicals used ...: M. Yanina Pepino et al., 'Sucralose affects glycemic and hormonal responses to an oral glucose load', *Diabetes Care*, 2013, vol. 36, no. 9, pp. 2530–35,

Page 66   In Australia, around 40 per cent of cattle ...: Food Standards Australia New Zealand, 'Hormonal growth promotants in beef', *FSANZ*, March 2011, foodstandards.gov.au/consumer/generalissues/hormonalgrowth/Pages/default.aspx

Page 69   ... a risk factor for breast cancer ...: Mark P.J. Vanderpump, 'The epidemiology of thyroid disease', *British Medical Bulletin*, 2011, vol. 99, no. 1, pp. 39–51.

Page 70   Research also points to a link ...: Giuseppe Carruba, 'Estrogen and prostate cancer: an eclipsed truth in an androgen-dominated scenario', *Journal of Cell Biochemistry*, 2007, vol. 102, no. 4. pp. 899–911.

PART 3: THE 28-DAY HORMONE REBALANCE

Preparing for the rebalance

Page 76   Naturally occurring hormones in some dairy products ...: Hassan Malekinejad & Aysa Rezabakhsh, 'Hormones in dairy foods and their impact on public health: a narrative review article', *Iranian Journal of Public Health*, 2015, vol. 44, no. 6, pp. 742–58.

Page 76   According to one study, women ...: Jennifer Lucero et al., 'Early follicular phase hormone levels in relation to patterns of alcohol, tobacco, and coffee use', *Fertility and Sterility*, 2001, vol. 76, no. 4, pp. 723–29.

Page 78   This method improves insulin resistance ...: T. Shiraev, 'Evidence based exercise – clinical benefits of high intensity interval training', *Australian Family Physician*, 2012, vol. 41. no. 12. pp. 960–62.

Page 78   Young vegetarian women ...: Brook Harmon et al., 'Oestrogen levels in serum and urine of vegetarian and omnivore premenopausal women', *Public Health Nutrition*, 2014, vol. 17, no. 9, pp. 2087–93.

Page 78   Another study suggests caffeine ...: Rebecca L Ferrini & Elizabeth Barrett-Connor, 'Caffeine intake and endogenous sex steroid levels in postmenopausal women: the Rancho Bernardo Study', *American Journal of Epidemiology*, 1996, vol. 144, no. 7, pp. 642–44.

Day 4: Love your liver

Page 113 Non-alcoholic fatty liver disease ...: S.A. Townsend & Philip N. Newsome, 'Non-alcoholic fatty liver disease in 2016', *British Medical Bulletin*, 2016, vol. 119, no. 1, pp. 143–56.

Day 6: Let's talk about our new favourite topic

Page 121 Those on a high-fibre diet ...: I.H. Ullrich & M.J. Albrink, 'The effect of dietary fiber and other factors on insulin response: role in obesity', *Journal of Environmental Pathology, Toxicology and Oncology*, 1985, vol. 5, no. 6, pp. 137–55.

Day 7: Give in

Page 125 He writes, 'The only thing ...': Eckhart Tolle, *The Power of Now: A Guide to Spiritual Enlightenment*, New World Library, Novato, California, 1997, p. 88.

Day 9: The link between stress, weight and hormones

Page 133 Chronically elevated cortisol levels ...: W.M. Jefferies, 'Cortisol and immunity', *Medical Hypotheses*, 1991, vol. 34, no. 3, pp. 198–208.

Day 10: Full-fat or skim?

Page 136 US nutritionist Walter Willett ...: Quoted in Jon White, 'Is full-fat milk best? The skinny on the dairy paradox', *New Scientist*, 21 February 2014.

Day 11: The importance of sleep

Page 140 When we sleep, we release melatonin ...: J. Hansen, 'Increased breast cancer risk among women who work predominantly at night', *Epidemiology*, 2001, vol. 12, no. 1, pp. 74–77.

Page 141 In one study, sleep-deprived women ...: Najib T. Ayas, 'A prospective study of self-reported sleep duration and incident diabetes in women', *Diabetes Care*, 2003, vol. 26, no. 2, pp. 380–84.

Day 12: How thirst affects cortisol

Page 145 ... water ... assists with weight reduction: Vinu A. Vij et al., 'Effect of "water induced thermogenesis" on body weight, body mass index and body composition of overweight subjects', *Journal of Clinical and Diagnostic Research*, 2013, vol. 7, no. 9, pp. 1894–96.

Day 13: The happy hormone, serotonin

Page 148 ... scientists are not sure if lower levels of serotonin ...: Benjamin D. Sachs et al., 'Brain 5-HT deficiency increases stress vulnerability and impairs antidepressant responses following psychosocial stress', *Proceedings of the National Academy of Sciences*, 2015, vol. 112, no. 8, pp. 2557–62.

Day 14: Emotional eating

Page 152 Women often overeat for emotional reasons ...: Valentina Vicennati et al., 'Stress-related development of obesity and cortisol in women', *Obesity (Silver Spring)*, 2009, vol. 17, no. 9, pp. 1678–83.

Page 153 In his book The Power of Habit ...: Charles Duhigg, *The Power of Habit: Why We Do What We Do in Life and Business*, Random House, New York, 2012, pp. 289–98.

Day 15: Try intermittent fasting

Page 157 Fasting has been shown to reduce oxidative stress ...: Martin P. Wegman, 'Practicality of intermittent fasting in humans and its effect on oxidative stress and genes related to aging and metabolism', *Rejuvenation Research*, 2015, vol. 18, no. 2, pp. 162–72.

Day 16: Acid overload, the thyroid and insulin levels

Page 160 Too much acidity in the body ...: William E. Mitch, 'Metabolic and clinical consequences of metabolic acidosis', *Journal of Nephrology*, 2006, vol.19, supplement 9, pp. S70–75.

Day 17: Are you starving by dinnertime?

Page 165 The US National Institute on Aging ...: Olga Carlson et al., 'Impact of reduced meal frequency without caloric restriction on glucose regulation in healthy, normal-weight middle-aged men and women', *Metabolism*, 2007, vol. 56, no. 12, pp. 1729–34.

Day 18: Coconut oil and insulin resistance

Page 169 Coconut oil is also high in lauric acid ...: Jon J. Kabara, 'Health oils from the tree of life: nutritional and health aspects of coconut oil', *Indian Coconut Journal*, 2003, vol. 31, pp. 2–8.

Page 169 Those fed the virgin coconut oil ...: Arunaksharan Narayanankutty et al., 'Virgin coconut oil maintains redox status and improves glycemic conditions in high fructose fed rats', *Journal of Food Science and Technology*, 2016, vol. 53, no. 1, pp. 895–901.

Page 169 Researchers from Sydney's Garvan Institute
...: Nigel Turner et al., 'Enhancement of muscle
mitochondrial oxidative capacity and alterations in
insulin action are lipid species-dependent: potent
tissue-specific effects of medium chain fatty acids',
Diabetes, 2009, vol. 58 no. 11, pp. 2547–54.

**Day 19: Are cortisol and insulin wreaking
havoc on your skin?**

Page 173 Fish – Filled with essential ...: P. Saldeen &
T. Saldeen, 'Women and omega-3 fatty acids',
Obstetrical and Gynecological Survey, 2004, vol.
59, no. 10, pp. 722–30, 745–46.

Day 22: Is MSG messing with your metabolism?

Page 185 In one study, people who consumed MSG ...:
Maeve Shannon et al., 'The endocrine disrupting
potential of monosodium glutamate (MSG) on
secretion of the glucagon-like peptide-1 (GLP-1) gut
hormone and GLP-1 receptor interaction',
Toxicology Letters, 2017, vol. 265, pp. 97–105.

Day 25: Insulin and soft drinks

Page 197 One study found that mice ...: Jotham Suez
et al., 'Artificial sweeteners induce glucose
intolerance by altering the gut microbiota', *Nature*,
2014, vol. 514, no. 7521, pp. 181–86.

Page 197 The Harvard School of Public Health ...: The
Nutrition Source, 'Soft drinks and disease', Harvard
T.H. Chan School of Public Health, n.d., hsph.harvard.
edu/nutritionsource/healthy-drinks/soft-drinks-
and-disease

Day 26: Candida and hormone chaos

Page 201 ... one factor affecting their trajectory is
hormones – particularly oestrogen ...: Georgina
Cheng et al., 'Cellular and molecular biology of
Candida albicans estrogen response', *Eukaryotic
Cell*, 2006, vol. 5, no. 1, pp. 180–91.

Day 27: Hormones and chronic inflammation

Page 205 When we consume too many sugars ...:
Dr Mercola, 'Fat for fuel: why dietary fat, not
glucose, is the preferred body fuel', *Peak Fitness*,
10 August 2012, fitness.mercola.com/sites/fitness/
archive/2012/08/10/fat-not-glucose.aspx

Page 205 One study found that drinking sugar-
sweetened beverages ...: Quanhe Yang et al., 'Added
sugar intake and cardiovascular diseases mortality
among US adults', *JAMA Internal Medicine*, 2014,
vol. 174, no. 4, pp. 516–24.

Page 205 A recent study found that high-fructose
corn syrup ...: L.R. DeChristopher, J. Uribarri & K.L.

Tucker, 'The link between soda intake and asthma:
science points to the high-fructose corn syrup, not
the preservatives: a commentary', *Nutrition and
Diabetes*, 2016, vol. 6, article no. e234.

RESOURCES

Nutritional supplements and food

Page 223 Magnesium: Up to 75 per cent of Australians
are estimated ...: David W. Killilea & Jeanette A.M.
Maier, 'A connection between magnesium deficiency
and aging: new insights from cellular studies',
Magnesium Research, 2008, vol. 21, no. 2, pp. 77–82.

Page 226 Herbs: Powerful anti-inflammatory and
insulin regulators: Wei-Jia Kong et al., 'Berberine
reduces insulin resistance through protein kinase
C-dependent up-regulation of insulin receptor
expression', *Metabolism*, 2009, vol. 58, no. 1,
pp. 109–19.

Acknowledgements

A massive thank you to our rockstar team at Pan Macmillan for this amazing experience. We are fortunate to collaborate with such talented, creative and dedicated people. Big thanks to Ingrid Ohlsson for her support, insights and sense of fun. To executive editor Virginia Birch for such a smooth and seamless ride. To creative manager Megan Pigott for nailing the book's atmospherics and design. To Nicola Young for forensic and thoughtful editing. To an incredible creative team – designer Sarah Odgers, photographer Cath Muscat and stylist Vanessa Austin. To expert food editor Rachel Carter. To Naomi van Groll for excellent wrangling. To brilliant publicist Yvonne Sewankambo. And to the super-efficient Roxarne Burns and Anna Ristevski.

Michele thanks her family – Steven, Gabi, Jake and Holly. Without them, nothing is sweet or in balance.

Jennifer thanks Jeff Forster, Catherine Fleming and Pat Fleming for excellent suggestions and support, and Anna-Louise Bouvier for the introduction to Michele.

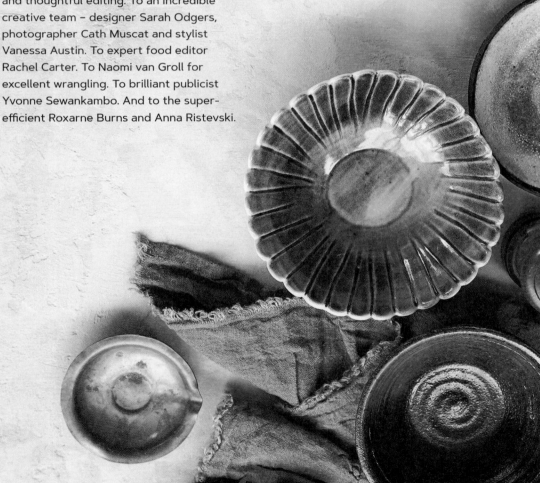

your notes:

INDEX

First published 2018 in Macmillan
by Pan Macmillan Australia Pty Limited
1 Market Street, Sydney, New South Wales
Australia 2000

A CIP catalogue record for this book is
available from the National Library of
Australia: http://catalogue.nla.gov.au

Design by Sarah Odgers
Photography by Cath Muscat
Prop and food styling by Vanessa Austin
Editing by Nicola Young and Rachel Carter
Props kindly supplied by Batch Ceramics,
   Katherine Mahoney Ceramics, Little White
   Dish, Chuchu and Thrown By Jo
Colour + reproduction by Splitting Image
   Colour Studio
Printed in China by 1010 Printing
   International Limited

We advise that the information contained
in this book does not negate personal
responsibility on the part of the reader
for their own health and safety. It is
recommended that individually tailored
advice is sought from your healthcare or
medical professional. The publishers and their
respective employees, agents and authors
are not liable for injuries or damage
occasioned to any person as a result of
reading or following the information
contained in this book.

10 9 8 7 6 5 4